Approaching Death

Approaching Death

A Companion's Guide to the End of Life

Renée Zeylmans

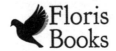

Floris Books

Translated by Philip Mees

Abridged from the Dutch *Stervensbegeleiding, een wederzijds proces*
First published in by Christofoor Publishers, Zeist in 2008
Second edition 2015
First published in English by Floris Books in 2019

British Library CIP Data available
ISBN 978-178250-603-4
Printed in Great Britain by Bell & Bain, Ltd

 Floris Books supports sustainable forest management by
printing this book on materials made from wood that comes
from responsible sources and reclaimed material

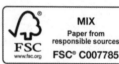

CONTENTS

Foreword – *Bastiaan Baan*   7

Preface   9

I Being a Companion to a Dying Person

1. Dying is Being Born in the Spiritual World   13
2. Death is as a Horizon   33
3. The 'Unknown' Hour of Death   45
4. Developing Awareness of Our Future Realm   55
5. When People Close to Us Die   65
6. The Person Dying as Fellow Traveller – *Monique van der Zanden* 75
7. When Young People Die   85
8. Experiences in a Children's Hospital – *Patricia de Vos*   93

II Care for the Dying

9. The Senses of the One Dying   109
10. The Language of Images at the Threshold – *Bert Voorhoeve* 125
11. Music for Terminally Ill People – *Hilly Bol*   131
12. Artistic Therapy – *Marieke Udo de Haes-Mulder*   141
13. External Therapy – *Pauli van Engelen* and *Toke Bezuijen* 147

III Death is Approaching

14. The Physiology of Dying – *Paul Schmitz, MD*   155
15. Euthanasia   159
16. Fasting until Death   165
17. The Double: My Shadow   167
18. The Moment of Dying   177

IV After Death

19. Coincidence?   185
20. The Funeral   191
21. Accompanying the Dying and Christian Ritual
    – *Bastiaan Baan*   197
22. Mourning by Friends and Relatives   205
23. Across the Threshold of Death   211
24. Staying Connected with the Dead   221

Afterword   235
Further Reading   237
Contributors   240

FOREWORD

Bastiaan Baan

As in a kaleidoscope this book presents a multi-coloured picture of accompanying the dying as a reciprocal process. You will find here the result of many views of this process in the light of various disciplines. It is well-known that the dying may have very different conversations with companions from different professions. Of course the themes discussed with physicians are not the same as those raised with a social worker or a pastor – let alone accompaniment based on various outlooks on life or religions.

And then there are the loving family members and friends who experience the dying process and the interaction with the dying person very differently than professional companions. Every one of the companions mentioned here sees a particular piece of the reality.

For Renée Zeylmans all these different views are valuable. In her courses – which I have in part given together with her for years – she respects every one of these views, particularly when it comes from another outlook on life than her own. Respect for everyone's freedom in this regard is of paramount importance to her.

Everyone who has met Renée Zeylmans in her work as caregiver, recognises besides this respectful attitude an almost inexhaustible will to help the other. With tremendous compassion she accompanies 'her people', as she calls them herself. Every connection becomes a reciprocal process that is frequently cultivated and developed over years.

This book is not only the result of a collection of different views and experiences; it is also the fruit of a 'life work': accompanying people dying and mourning, and those who have died.

PREFACE

For a year I wrestled to put into words what in fact cannot be reduced to words: the process every one of us has to go through when we are confronted with suffering, leave-taking, dying, the hope of a new birth in the spiritual world.

How do we accompany the dying? And how do they accompany us? What can we give them? And what do they give us?

No two people are the same, and so every dying process is individual. For this reason you will not find any methodologies or theories in this book. A nurse who followed one of my courses in accompanying the dying and mourning said afterwards: 'I expected to be able to learn a lot here, but now I realise that I actually have to unlearn a lot.'

I wanted to write a book with experiences that might enrich the reader, that sometimes throw a different light on things, evoke recognition, console, reach out; a book that leaves room for different choices. A book with practical information reaching across the threshold of death, but also with contemplations and points of view from various outlooks on life and cultures. My motto was: 'What I don't know or see need not be untrue.' This has helped me to be open-minded.

I have written this book for professionals and volunteers in care-giving situations, but also for those who are close to, or immediately involved with, the death of a loved one.

The basis of the decision to act or not to act is for me always love. The most important aspect in the encounter between two persons is, in my view, your ability to put yourself in the place of the other. When we have the courage to look our own death in the face, we can have the courage to put ourselves in the place of a dying person. That makes us into a companion.

Fortunately I was not alone during all these months while I wrestled with this subject. I also had companions, even angels, on my path. I felt carried by those living around me and by those who had died and from whom I had had to take leave. Many people made valuable contributions, often consisting of the most personal experiences, valuable knowledge, and life wisdom. They helped in the creation of this book. They all had the inner urge to give. I hope that their love may resound through these pages, and that it may become consolation and relief on the difficult journey made by the dying and their companions, and open a perspective for them that reaches across the horizon.

For us, living human beings, the dead may perhaps seem far away. But they are here around us, in our future realm, indissolubly connected with the here and now.

I

BEING A COMPANION TO A DYING PERSON

The idea of the transience
Of all earthly things
Is a source of boundless suffering,
And a source of boundless consolation.

Maria von Ebner-Eschenbach (1830–1916)

1

DYING IS BEING BORN IN THE SPIRITUAL WORLD

Just as one throws out old clothes
And then takes on other, new ones,
So the embodied self casts out old bodies
As it gets other, new ones.

The Bhagavad Gita, 2.22

If we are present at the birth of a child, we may have a feeling of a border or threshold experience. We momentarily sense the spiritual world the child came from. We see it colouring rosy at the first breath, the umbilical cord is cut, and then we know that the child has become a citizen of the earth. At the time of dying too, an 'umbilical cord' is cut. In the Bible this is called the 'silver cord' (Eccl 12:6).

In former times the spiritual world was a reality for people. We come from it and return to it. Birth was a leave-taking from the spiritual world and a joyous welcome on earth. Conversely, dying was a leave-taking on earth and a joyous reunion in the spiritual world.

A Jewish legend relates:

When the Neshamah [the soul dwelling with God] has seen everything in heaven, and when it experiences the height of bliss, then the angel announces that the moment of birth is approaching. Fear descends on the Neshamah, dread of what is coming. Entry into the world of form announces itself. The angel then says that he will leave the Neshamah alone. But the angel also says that at the end of the way through the world of exile, which begins with birth, he will be there again to take the Neshamah home. The first cry of the child is the cry of distress of the Neshamah when she suddenly feels abandoned.

The child that is born goes through the 'eye of the needle', coming out of timeless space. The death of a human being is as a birth, but in the reverse direction. At birth we are very alert, we have all we need 'in stock.' But what do we have in stock for the process of dying? How do you connect with the true being of a person who is dying, who is wrestling in an agony of death, wrestling to make it through the eye of the needle? How can you have a conversation without words?

When a loved one dies you know him or her very well. But if you are a physician, nurse or companion sitting at the sick-bed of a person who is dying, you have to admit that you know very little about this human being, about the spiritual being that has lived in that body, and that is now in a process of finding a way of connecting with its essential core in some manner. Perhaps there is a patient history available and we know something of the background of this person. But who is wrestling there, we don't really know. That being is still hidden in the bodily enclosure, but it loosens itself more and more. We can actually see in a dying human being also how 'naked' someone can be in such a moment, how vulnerable they are.

It is a real art to accompany a dying person in just the right way. We have to learn to watch with different eyes by not only focusing on the event of the dying itself, and on what we have to do or ought to do in that regard. By strengthening our observation we can develop a sense of what the patient needs without them even asking for it. If there is physical pain we can begin to perceive that the patient also suffers from other pains.

In all interventions you might want to make, the first consideration is to create room to enter into a connection with the patient, so that reciprocal action is preserved.

When my mother was dying (aged 99), she was quite rebellious. Mother was vexed, angry and afraid. Rightfully so. She had been made a victim of a practice of abstinence, and the horror that came over her when she became aware of it was deeply moving. I could actually not do very much for her, and the care in the home for the elderly was hard and efficient. A day before her death she was still put in the shower to wash her hair that, because of my efforts with lavender oil, had become somewhat greasy. They also brought her 'sociably' to the day room.

When subsequently she was lying in her room again I read to her a few random passages from a book that was very dear to her and of which she had beautiful memories. I thoroughly enjoyed reading these texts to her – in these improvised situations the right fragments jump out all by themselves. When I stopped reading my mother nodded in agreement, in other words, not in dismissal, and the fact that she reacted was in itself remarkable. 'Funny,' she squeaked. Knowing my mother I took this as a sign that she had certainly taken something in and understood it.

I decided to go home briefly and come back in the evening. During dinner at home I discussed the situation with my husband and sons. In addition to being a mother, she had also been a violinist and had played in quartets with friends. Once when a friend of mine died she had said to me that she did not understand why there was no beautiful music being played at the deathbed. That went against my grain at the time because I was convinced that music had to be real, played live at a deathbed. Now it suddenly came back to me. So, I quickly found a little cassette recorder with two tapes and hurried to the deathbed.

Mother was lying on her side and did not look up. Fortunately it was remarkably quiet in the home. The patients were in bed, and the staff were drinking coffee far away from us at the end of a hallway. I began very softly with the *Stabat Mater* by Pergolesi. After I had also played the *Rosamunde Quartet* by Schubert, I started to feel moved myself, and also felt compassion for this life that had such a difficult time coming to an end. I switched the player off, walked to Mother's bed and sat down on a chair to have a good look at her. While I was doing this she suddenly sat up, opened a pair of bright blue eyes, looked at me, waited a little, and died – the music still soundlessly around us.

– Tientje Huismans

Striving to work together

When a person dies they do this not just physically and psychically, but also socially. The dying person comes into a process in which they withdraw, so to speak, from the social context that exists for us as long as we live here on earth. Then they have to take a 'leap' into another context, the social context of the spiritual world.

According to people who have had a near death experience, the dead are received over there at their birth into the heavenly spheres by people who have previously died. This means that what happens does not solely depend on us as companions. Perhaps it is actually true that a number of souls are standing around the one who is dying, souls we cannot see but are all active helping the dying person from their side. Wouldn't it therefore be wonderful to work together with them?

From caregiver to companion

Being a companion of a dying person means that I feel the distress, suffering and joy of the other as if it were my own. Then a bridge is built within me that we can stand on together.

The ability to be a companion does not begin at the deathbed, but in daily life, and it has everything to do with the way we interact with our fellow human beings. For how can we be a support for a dying person if we have not, at least to some extent, acquired the approach of a companion in daily life? It is also related to the way we ourselves handle crisis, grief and joy in life. For doesn't every change, every crisis we go through, carry death and resurrection in itself?

Dying people find themselves in the greatest crisis of their life, a crisis that comes with confusing and violent emotions, and is greater than they can probably put into words themselves. As a caregiver, you are deeply involved in this crisis.

In such situations it is important that you have the courage to practise self-reflection every time, for you inevitably also go through a process, no matter how experienced you are. If you don't want to do this, or don't have the courage to face yourself, it is good to make that conscious, for it always influences your behaviour and actions in relation to the dying. They hear in the sound of your voice whether you are willing to carry them inwardly and are ready for the confrontation. What counts is that you truly connect with them. This is not a path of the head, but one of the heart. 'Only with the heart can you see well,' said the fox in *The Little Prince* by Antoine de Saint Exupéry. Actions performed merely out of a methodology or routine cannot remain hidden from the dying, for their consciousness is broader and more intuitive than ours.

In training we are often told to keep a distance, the so-called professional approach, and we are taught all kinds of methods for this. But are there still people who want this kind of caregiving? People today see right through those things. We want to meet a person with a loving, listening ear, in brief, a companion who walks with us on our way.

Martin Buber relates a story of the Hasidic Rabbi of Sasor who, when he saw someone suffer, had such compassion that he made that person's suffering his own. When he was asked how that is possible, he replied: 'What, com-passion? Isn't that suffering-together-with? How can I do differently than make it my own?' Dostoevsky speaks in all his works of this com-passion, this suffering-together-with the suffering of the other: 'If we experience the brother creature in him, we can do no other.'

If we learn how to deal with our emotions, a mutual connection will grow, and sharing joys and sorrows will bestow life wisdom on us. Being a companion does not mean drowning in emotions, but discerning and accompanying the deeper layer of grief. Repressing feelings or hiding behind a professional attitude will lead sooner to burnout than if you face them and work them through. By practising such a professional attitude for a longer time you harm yourself, and this inevitably leads to exhaustion, sometimes only many years later.

Those dying also don't ask us to pour our wisdom all over them. Assisting those dying means a closeness, but also a distance.

> It frequently happens when you visit someone who has a chronic or terminal illness to comfort or help them, that after leaving you feel comforted or helped yourself. You notice then that these people have become so wise and mild in the course of their illness that they radiate something into the world. The inner struggle that they go through because of the illness is not lost when they die; they take it with them as strength through the gate of death.
> – Joop van Dam, physician

Let us make sure that a person in distress is not forced to listen to our grief and worries, so that those who need consolation, often radiating a kind of receptivity, do not in fact have to hear the troubles of someone else. This is a trap that we can also face in daily life; may I burden the other with my feelings that arise at the deathbed? (See also Chapter 5.)

It does not mean that there can be no mutual exchange. You participate in the joys and sorrows of the dying person – a laugh and a tear. But what comes up in you needs to be weighed to determine whether it contributes something to the other. Holding back what came up in you is then borne with dignity, and you have to look for a way in yourself to work it through. You put it in a place where it can ripen, until the moment comes when it can bear fruit for the future.

That is the gift of the dying. Not just trouble and pain, but also growth and blossoming.

How do I come across?

A deep feeling of loneliness can grow in a dying person when we come in like a bull in a china shop without any feeling for their state of consciousness and the different reality they are gradually entering. Too often when we visit a dying or sick person we come in like a whirlwind, full of life and optimism that really doesn't correspond with the patient's phase of life. Don't exhibit all your power of life; you overwhelm the other with it, and it can be critical.

Just as an exercise, pay some attention to how people come into your house. One will, in a manner of speaking, immediately fill the whole room and is strongly present. Another slips in modestly, doesn't take any space and most of the time is a good listener. Hold back, therefore, make yourself 'thinner.' You can actually practise this while you are on your way to the visit, by focusing your thoughts on the patient and putting away everything else that is in your mind. In this way you make space for the other to enter into you.

This does not mean that we have to be sombre. I have experienced a fine humour at deathbeds and from stories of surviving relatives. Truly good humour is vanquished pain.

> A dying woman asked her nurse, 'What is the name of your daughter?'
> 'Lena.'
> 'My chicken is also called Lena.' And then she died.

Listening, communication at the deathbed

How intensely can we listen to a dying person? Are we capable of listening in such a way that we are all ears, all attention, that we are totally present? During life, we experience how important it is, if we sit speaking with someone, to feel we are met with undivided attention. If we give undivided attention to the other, we have done what is most important. Truly listening means becoming inwardly silent. Hearing always means being absorbed in the other. Speaking from heart to heart is love without compulsion or urgency.

Try also to listen 'between the lines.' If a terminally ill person likes to have the television on, this can be a normal wish, but it could also be for an unspoken reason with an underlying message. Perhaps they are fearful, lacking the courage to talk, and try to fill the silence with the television.

> The reality of the other does not lie in what he reveals to you,
> but in what he cannot reveal to you. When therefore you want
> to understand him, do not listen to what he says, but rather to
> what he conceals.
> – *Kahlil Gibran,* The Prophet

In caregiving, sitting across from someone and really becoming inwardly silent is very difficult. To practise inner hearing we have to create space in ourselves. Whenever someone starts to speak, all too frequently a judgment rises up in us right away. We feel sympathy or antipathy and actually wish that the other would become a little different. As a result, we become unable to really listen and we don't truly see the other; we are often continually busy with what the other evokes in us and, as a result, we react subjectively. Often this is caused by our own memories and experiences that are called up in us. Dying people perceive this. They are not heard, and stop speaking. In caregiving self-reflection is important. Listening is an intensive path of schooling.

A big stumbling block is that we often have a feeling that we have to do something when we visit a dying person. It is as if we cannot sit still and simply listen; listen on different levels. For such a person may not say a word, but speak volumes. Can we already do something by just being there? How are we present?

The Talmud says that it is considered a deed of great charity to sit with a dying person so that their soul is supported in its transition by a soul in a peaceful condition. What determines the quality of companionship to those dying is not intervention, but simple presence.

Speaking out of observing and listening to the other creates an encounter from which something new can arise. Person to person meetings thus make it possible to create value in the last phase of life.

Pitfalls

If we have the privilege of being present at someone's death we are perhaps faced with a greater task than the path of schooling that is part of everyday life. Impatience is a pitfall. Out of impatience we could, even with the best of intentions, make bad decisions. At a deathbed we often have to have incredible patience. Just like birth, dying takes time. As a relative you might catch yourself thinking: how much longer? Once when that happened to me I was deeply ashamed; I felt how small I really was as a human being. But because we become tired, it is only human that we long for the end – on behalf of the dying, but also the bystanders. Our stamina is put to the test because our whole society is so solution-oriented.

Helping gives satisfaction, strengthening our sense of self-worth. Receiving, on the other hand, makes us vulnerable because we are confronted with ourselves. The urge to help may come from hidden egoism or desire. Enthusiasm may therefore also be a pitfall, especially if it expresses itself in a desire to do something, to be active. We are trapped in the idea that concern and activity are inseparable, but a repeated feeling of wanting to help a dying person is perhaps the right attitude. This inner urge is a gift. A gift creates no responsibility for the receiver! Giving unconditional love does not ask for a reward, but is a human duty. In the end, the reward may be that the dying person gives you gifts that increase your life wisdom. Frequently we realise only much later that, exactly by being present at the process of dying, we have learned more about the mystery of life. Who then accompanies whom? That is something I have often wondered about.

Finding balance in accompanying the dying

But as companion, you also need protection yourself. I certainly do not underestimate the strength, courage and stamina that is demanded. Developing an inner approach that sharpens your intuition could be of great help. With this in mind I quote below what Bastiaan Baan taught in my course on accompanying dying and mourning people.

> When Chagall painted the appearance of the spiritual world in the world of humans, in the form of three angel figures with Abraham, he used an original and significant way of representing the angel world. If you look at the feet of the

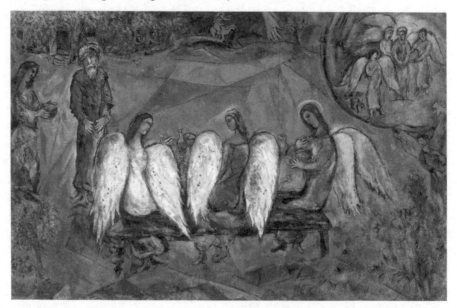

Marc Chagall, Abraham and the Three Angels, *Musée national du message biblique Marc-Chagall, Nice, France.*

angels you see something remarkable. For in his picture Chagall followed an old icon tradition by showing them with one bare foot and one shod foot. We witness an element here that is precious for our caregiving: you have to approach a dying person with one bare and one shod foot. This means that you come with part of your being – openness, receptivity and vulnerability – as if barefoot. For instance, think of that very difficult patient who cannot and will not depart and shuts themselves up in their unbelief. There all your senses are open and you have made a clean slate of yourself to enter into an encounter with that person again and again.

But be warned! Another part of yourself must be shod, has to be covered and has to be prepared for obstacles and obstruction that can trip you up. Therefore: open and closed, vulnerable and strong, receptive and active, giving space and taking space. That is the balance you somehow have to create so you can both accompany the dying in the right way and also remain intact yourself.

The well-known problem of hospice workers and nurses is that they become burned out by their care for the dying who, unbeknownst to themselves, suck the living dry. You have to be prepared for that; you can become exhausted if, to use Chagall's picture again, you enter only 'barefoot'.

The trick – and this is an important point of preparation – is to find the right balance before you enter the room of the dying person. Balance is not just a noun or a verb; it is an art. It is a continual movement on the balance beam. When we stand upright, without being aware of it, we are constantly adjusting our balance. Physicians and physical therapists know that. It looks as if we are standing still, but is a precarious balance. All the time we need to correct ourselves to find the balance between the extremes of left and right, front and back, high and low. More than on any other occasion in our accompaniment of the dying we need such an inner capacity. While at all times focusing on what is happening with the dying person, we need at the same time to stay aware of ourselves and, if the moment arises, be prepared to open wide the door so we can be totally there for the other. But if we sense that we lack the necessary forces or feel an impure element coming in, we need to be able to close the door again.

There is a religious expression for this in the Book of Revelation, in the letter to the Philadelphians. Those words show that this is not only a capacity we have to conquer step by step, but also one that is bestowed on us by Christ. In the letter to Philadelphia this is indicated with the words: 'These are the words of him who is holy and true, who holds the key of David. What he opens no one can shut, and what he shuts no one can open' (Rev 3:7).

Such a key is what we need in every form of caregiving, every form of encounter. But unfortunately we often don't possess that kind of key. Just look at caregiving and at the way you meet other people. If you only open wide the door, you eventually lose yourself; if you only keep the door closed, nothing happens in interaction. You need this 'key of David,' the key that opens what no one can shut. The moment I open the door of my closed personality there is no longer any obstacle to entering in. I open it as a sovereign act. The moment I am being asked too much or I sense that clouded elements are coming in, I close the door so that I remain standing and the other does not have the opportunity to unload negativism on me or take advantage of me. That is the crucial point that enables you in every form of caregiving to find the right balance between giving and taking.

Fear: confronting yourself

> We tend to think that courageous people are not afraid of
> anything. In actual fact, they are intimately familiar with fear.
> – *Pema Chödrön*

Accompanying the dying can become a hard confrontation with ourselves and with the question of the meaning of life. But the insight this enables us to acquire is a great gift, even if to receive it we often have to go through hell.

When we are close to a dying person we become more or less conscious of what usually remains unconscious, namely our own mortality. We realise that what the dying person is going through will also happen to us one day. Because of this we not only have to deal with the fear of the one dying, who is losing their sense of physical security, but also with our own fear. Being confronted with a dying person brings our deepest fears to the surface.

Avoiding those fears is senseless; we will have to come to terms with them. Our recognition of our own fears around death will help us understand the fears of the dying. Only if we face this fear can it subside. Recognised fear loses its threatening power over us.

> One of the principal reasons why we are so afraid of death is that we ignore the reality of transience. We always view change as loss and suffering. And when it occurs, we try to numb ourselves as much as possible. We gratuitously and obstinately assume that durability gives us security, and transience does not. But we simply have to get used to the idea of transience.
> – *Sogyal Rinpoche*, Glimpse after Glimpse

Everything we are not able to command and control, the unexpected or the unknown, can cause fear. In fear we lose our solid ground, our self-awareness is undermined. In fear the blood drains out of our skin, out of the periphery back into the centre; we turn pale. Fear is often visible on the outside, even in our gestures. We clasp our head or our heart as if to protect it. We shrink as if we want to hide. In brief, in fear we look for support within ourselves.

These days people see the value again of swaddling babies, which in prior times was common. With this you create a boundary which the baby cannot yet give itself. It creates peace and security. We can also experience that in the process of dying. The spirit, our immortal I, begins to leave the physical body. Those dying lose the security of the body. That may cause fear, and in that situation a boundary may feel good, such as a pillow on both sides or at the feet. Most of all, we can 'swaddle' the dying in our unconditional love.

If you dare walk to the wall of your fear, you will see that it is a portal.

Fear is not only negative. It protects us, for instance, from overly impulsive steps. It can make us attentive, such as in traffic. Attentiveness is a capacity born from fear. By looking fear in the eye, taking it seriously and working it through, we can build up a positive inner attitude to cope with a situation. When fear is transformed courage arises, and courage is a feeling that fills us with strength.

Fear and courage can keep each other in balance. This gives us the strength to take on the exacting task of standing by a dying person, and it also protects us from an urge to perform. Being lovingly present out of the depths of our heart also gives us the strength to confront our fear.

Love: a force that breaks through the boundary of death

You can mean something for another if you have the courage to co-experience their fear. Not only their fear of death, of taking leave, of pain and dependence, loss of control and discouragement, but also the fear that life may have been meaningless.

It is important to strengthen these forces of courage and love by prayer and conscious inner schooling. In prayer we address the divine spark in us and call on forces to help us take the right road. Anja experienced how her dying sister-in-law screamed in fear:

> It was November 1993. I was sitting by the head of the bed.
> Joyce was lying in a hospital bed close to the window of her
> room. Next to her stood a little table with two candles, a bible

and a little incense. Joyce was very restless, tossed and turned, and called out all day long. She shouted all the time: 'Mom, help me, help me!' and my mother-in-law could no longer bear it. When I tried to talk to Joyce she did not react, I could not reach her anymore. I proposed to my mother-in-law to say the Lord's Prayer aloud together; we did it irrespective of the shouting. I knew that Joyce had a connection with this prayer. During the last line of the prayer she briefly stopped shouting and said the line with us. We decided to repeat the prayer a number of times, and in so doing I experienced, and was astonished by, the power of this prayer. As soon as we stopped, Joyce started to shout again. My mother-in-law sat down beside the bed, and I suggested calling Joyce's children. We continued the prayer until she became quiet again and the shouting stopped. The next morning she died peacefully.

The way of Artaban, the Fourth Wise Man

What can we do in a situation when someone is dying and we have the urge to do something? We can fix everything in a list, meaning that we prescribe what steps have to be taken and we know precisely what to do and when. But before you know it, it is the list that determines what you do, and the connection with the patient is gone. You give something to ease pain, but the person doesn't only have pain, they are in a process in which, among other things, pain plays an important role.

In the story about Artaban, *The Story of the Other Wise Man*, Henry van Dyke indicates a way we might follow as companion of a dying person. Artaban is a friend of the three kings, Melchior, Balthazar and Caspar. All four of them have seen the star appear in heaven which told them that the King of Kings was born. They want to go to him to bring him gifts. The three kings go ahead, Artaban will join them later.

Artaban sells all his possessions and with the proceeds he buys a sapphire, a ruby and a pearl; the three gifts he wants to give to the King of Kings. He starts his journey, but is too late, the caravan of the three kings has already left. When he reaches Bethlehem on his own, the holy family with the child has also disappeared. Artaban the Magian does not give up, he continues his search. During his journey he repeatedly encounters people who are in distress and, with pain in his heart, he uses the gifts he has brought for the King of Kings to help his fellow human beings. Finally, after 33 years, he arrives in Jerusalem, exhausted and ready to die, but still looking for his King. He has one gift left.

A troop of Macedonian soldiers came down the street, dragging a young girl with torn dress and dishevelled hair. As the Magian paused to look at her with compassion, she broke suddenly from the hands of her tormentors and threw herself at his feet, clasping him around the knees...

'Have pity on me,' she cried, 'and save me!' ...

He took the pearl from his bosom. Never had it seemed so luminous, so radiant, so full of tender, shining lustre. He laid it in the hand of the slave.

'This is thy ransom, daughter! It is the last of my treasures which I kept for the King.'

While he spoke, the darkness of the sky thickened, and shuddering tremors ran through the earth, heaving convulsively like the breast of one who struggles with mighty grief...

What had he to fear? What had he to live for? He had given away the last remnant of his tribute for the King. He had parted with the last hope of finding Him. The quest was over, and it had failed. But even in that thought, accepted and embraced, there was peace. It was not submission. It was something more profound and searching. He knew that all was well, because he had done the best that he could, from day to day. He had been true to the light that had been given to him. He had looked for more. And if he had not found it, if a failure was all that came out of his life, doubtless that was the best that was possible.

He had not seen the revelation of 'life everlasting, incorruptible, and immortal.' But he knew that if he could live his life over again, it could not be otherwise than it had been.

One more lingering pulsation of the earthquake quivered through the ground. A heavy tile, shaken from the roof, fell and struck the old man on the temple. He lay breathless and pale, with his grey head resting on the girl's shoulder, and blood trickling from the wound. As she bent over him, fearing that he was dead, there came a voice through the twilight, very small and still, like music sounding from a distance, in which the notes are clear but the words are lost. The girl turned to see if someone had spoken from the window above them, but she saw no one.

Then the old man's lips began to move, as if in answer, and she heard him say in the Parthian tongue:

'Not so, my Lord. For when did I see thee hungry and fed thee? Or thirsty and gave thee drink? When did I see thee a stranger, and took thee in? Or naked, and clothed thee? When did I see thee sick or in prison, and came to thee? Three-and-thirty years have I looked for thee; but I have never seen thy face, nor ministered to thee, my King.'

He ceased, and the sweet voice came again. And again the maid heard it, very faintly and far away. But now it seemed as though she understood the words: 'Truly, I say to you, inasmuch as you have done it unto the least of these my brethren, you have done it unto me.'

A calm radiance of wonder and joy lighted the pale face of Artaban like the first ray of dawn on a snowy mountain-peak. One long, last breath of relief exhaled gently from his lips.

His journey was ended. His treasures were accepted. The Other Wise Man had found the King.

Artaban's way is the way which I think the dying human being needs. It is a way that teaches how you can mobilise the love in yourself for the suffering human being, for the dying person is all too often also a suffering human being. When you are dying you have to completely surrender yourself, without always being understood or heard, or without people with whom you can share what you are going through.

Artaban gave everything away that he had wanted to give to the King of Kings. Out of love he gave his sapphire, ruby and pearl to people who were suffering.

We all have gifts. We all have something in us that is unique and that we can give to the dying. If I follow the rules and administer a painkiller, it is no gift, for we had worked that out and agreed it together to avoid mistakes; it doesn't come from my heart. But I can imagine that the painkiller does become a gift at the moment when I administer it: I can mobilise my love, I can engage my inner being in what I do.

In so doing I need to listen very carefully to what the dying person needs, so that I truly hear them. Artaban did not scatter his things at random. If we are particularly touched by a dying person we might do that, but it would not be right; there has to be an interaction, a breathing process. The flow between the dying one and us has to be in continual movement.

But what is that movement? We can sit down and pay attention to what is happening. We can wait and see if a moment comes when something has to be done. But we can also try to come into movement inwardly. If I move inwardly I can, as it were, with my life forces help carry what is taking place in the ill, dying person. For this I have to know what this person is going through. Artaban's way teaches us to give the dying person what they need.

Contemplation: Positive thinking

I often think of consolation. And now I am musing: what is
no consolation? I often run into people who bandy the term
'positive thinking' about as if it were a cure-all. In its own
right, a positive attitude in life and in your own life situation
is of course fine. When I was twenty I read Robert Peale's
book *Positive Thinking* and it was an eye-opener. But should
we impose this attitude on another person? And if we want to
encourage people to approach something in a positive manner,
do we do it subtly enough? If not, we may hurt them; it may
sound like a condemnation that they are thinking negatively.

I witnessed that with a mother and daughter. The mother
had an incurable illness and was expected to die soon. The
daughter was unable to resign herself to this, feeling that her
mother had to think positively, then miracles could happen.
The mother had already accepted her approaching death and
knew that there was no escaping it.

The difficulty did not lie in the process of the mother, but
in that of the daughter who was unable to accept and work with
the idea of approaching death. For both it was a difficult path
with many reproaches: 'If you really loved me you would fight
for your life.'

Can we find consolation in people who give a positive twist
to every expression of impotence and grief? They can give you
the feeling that you are falling short and are complaining. But
accepting what is happening to you is also a form of positive
thinking!

2

DEATH IS AS A HORIZON

Death is as a horizon
And a horizon is merely
A limitation of our sight.

When you hear that the time you have left to live is limited, it can be a big shock. Suddenly everything is relative – everything you believe in and is important to you, your goals and your striving. Your whole value system has to go back to the drawing board. We all have methods we use for avoidance, to fool ourselves, evade confrontational events, and avoid self-knowledge. We often think: Later, not now. But then suddenly there is no later anymore; the process of dying sets in.

The past rises up in you, as it were, and flashes of present and future thrust themselves into your consciousness. You might still be able to evade the confrontation, but deep down you know that there is no way back anymore. Thus you find old pain, unprocessed grief, maybe events and experiences you had pushed from your memory. Emotions emerge about the life that was lived on earth and the inevitable in prospect. Are you able to face it? You will have to grow toward it, and that often involves denial. I prefer calling denial a salutary anaesthesia. Realising that you are going to die is too huge, too confrontational to comprehend right away. Slowly but surely you get the opportunity to take your life into your own hands once again. Will you go through it or around it? Are you able to look yourself and your life in the eye? You remain autonomous; out of your own free will you decide how to stand in the circumstances of your life.

Those near the one who is going to die also go through a similar process.

> He who is aware of inconstancy
> And likewise realises that existence as a human being
> Offers immense potential,
> Appreciates that he has no time to lose.
> – *Dalai Lama,* Open Heart, Clear Mind

During our whole life we are subject to death. Our body goes through continual dying processes from the time of our birth. When we are young it is not yet so visible because the vitality and constructive forces that oppose this are still strong. But as we age, the death processes in our body gradually begin to dominate. The continual process of breakdown and renewal, which alternately take place during waking and sleeping, is the fundamental ground of our existence.

The same is true for our inner world of experience. There also we witness repeated movements downward and upward, pulling back and growing. Developing awareness of this process is a path of learning on which dying and death find a place in our lives as someone we know, like a friend. Thus we can grow toward the final moment of dying.

What is dying? The simple way of answering that question might be 'being dead,' or 'passed on.' The latter term is perhaps closest to reality: passing on to another form of being, to another form of living.

When someone dies, the body remains behind. But what happens to the vitality that had offset the continual dying processes mentioned above? And to the inner world of thoughts and images?

A fourfold image of the human being

In this book we will frequently encounter the image of the fourfold human being as described in anthroposophy and other places. It is an ancient image; the great theologian Origen (*c.* 185–254) already used it, as did Church Father Augustine (354–430). In the course of time this picture became eroded. At the Council of Constantinople in the ninth century the spirit was abolished by the Church, and in the nineteenth century the soul was abolished by science.

The fourfold human image distinguishes four parts of the human being:

The *physical body*: our outwardly visible body.

The *etheric body*, *ether body* or *life body*: the life body that surrounds our physical body; it has to do with creating form and growth, thinking and remembering.

The *astral body*, also called *soul* or *psyche*: this is where our soul life manifests.

The *I* or *self*: our individuality. We are the only ones who can say to this: I am.

The physical body

Our physical body is the outer 'instrument,' our clothing of flesh. In it our immortal 'I' can manifest as an individual being. Living in a body means we are separate from every other human being or object. The element of space means that we exist in a state of separateness. I am sitting here, there sits someone else; we look at each other, we sense a distance, a contrast. In our body we stand over against the other. In space we are always separated from each other. But because of our I, which inhabits our body, we can take a standpoint. What wants to come into development needs space!

Then Almitra spoke again and said,
And what of marriage, Master?
And he answered saying:
You were born together, and together you shall be forevermore.
You shall be together when the white wings of death scatter your days.

Ay, you shall be together even in the silent memory of God.
But let there be spaces in your togetherness,
And let the winds of the heavens dance between you.
Love one another, but make not a bond of love:
Let it rather be a moving sea between the shores of your souls.
Fill each other's cup but drink not from one cup.
Give one another of your bread but eat not from the same loaf.
Sing and dance together and be joyous, but let each one of you
be alone,
Even as the strings of a lute are alone though they quiver with
the same music.
Give your hearts, but not into each other's keeping,
For only the hand of life can contain your hearts.
And stand together, yet not too near together;
For the pillars of the temple stand apart,
And the oak tree and the cypress grow not in each other's shadow.
– *Kahlil Gibran*, The Prophet

The life body or ether body

The life body (or body of formative forces) penetrates deeply into the physical body and causes it to grow and develop. Part of the essence of the life body is the task to protect the physical body at all times from decomposition. The physical body is permeated by life forces, forces that see to it that the body can grow, can restore itself in case of injuries, has the capacity to regenerate. These forces also give it vitality.

In the first years of life the life body uses all its forces for the further forming of the physical body, which is not complete at birth. Around the seventh year those up-building processes are complete; part of the life body is freed for consciousness. You could call this the birth of the life body. The life forces can become mobilised for real thinking by the child. As a result, children around age seven (the time of the change of teeth) begin to observe the world differently.

Mom, do people see the world the way I see it?
– *Joram, age 7*

The life body surrounds the physical body; it is connected to it by a silver cord, as it were, just as the umbilical cord connects the embryo with the mother. During sleep this connection is still completely intact; in a near-death experience it is almost broken. But when it breaks, the life body separates from the physical body and death sets in. From ancient times, esoteric tradition has connected the moon sphere with the element of silver; hence the name 'silver cord'.

As my father was approaching his death I experienced that dying is a transition from this world to another world, connected by a cord. My father tried to cut this cord. One afternoon my mother and I were visiting him. My father was restless; with his fingers he was making a movement as if snipping something off. My mother and I could not understand what he was doing. The next day he told my mother the following:

'I was in a light, love-filled world where, by the way, I was most welcome. I wanted very much to go there, but I had not yet taken leave of you. That made me sad. I also saw that I was connected by a silver cord with the world in which I am connected with you. And yet I wanted to cut this cord, but I couldn't do it. Slowly I fell back, and now I am with you so I can take leave of you.'

Full of thankfulness and joy my father then took us in his arms, and a few days later he died.
– *Marieke*

The life body contains our memories, the pictures we have formed for ourselves. When the life body lets go of the physical body after death, these memories manifest in the life panorama, where time becomes space, and which unrolls like a scroll, as described in the Book of Revelation.

The 'film of life'

Jewish wise men report that each of us, shortly after our death, experience how our entire past life passes in front of us, while we account for all our deeds, words, feelings and thoughts. According to rabbinical literature, these images take the form of a panorama, a very fast, three-dimensional overview of the important scenes and moments in our life, both the good and the bad, in overwhelmingly bright colours. Every detail of the experiences gained in this life is shown to us. It is as if we can review our entire life at a glance ... The rabbis say about this: 'At the hour of his departure to his eternal home all his deeds are shown him, and then the angels say to him: "On such and such a day you did or said this or that".'

The soul then understands the reasons and consequences of all her thoughts, words, feelings and deeds. The events are placed in perspective to each other. We see the effect our behaviour had on others, also strangers. We begin to understand how much the lives of all human beings are related to each other ... An angel has been appointed to each human being, and every day he notes what the person has done, so that everything he does is known to the Blessed Holy One. Everything is written in the chronicle of his life and authenticated with a seal.

– *Lewis Solomon,* The Jewish Book of Living and Dying

The soul (astral body)

The word 'astral' comes from the Latin *aster* or *astrum*, both meaning star. The astral body is the member of our being that encloses the life body. It is also called soul body.

A plant has a physical body and a life body just as we do. In plants too, all kinds of life processes take place. But differently from plants, we are able to have inner experiences and sensations; we can have hunger and thirst, sorrow, pain, love – in brief, experiences in our soul. Everything we feel, our thoughts, everything that moves us in our life we take into our soul, into our soul body, where we become aware of it. Thus in the soul body work all human passions, desires and urges, as well as our sense impressions.

Until puberty the forces of the astral body work for the development of our sense organs and our musculature. Around age fourteen another far-reaching change takes place. The soul body becomes free for consciousness, so that the capacity of our independent thinking, feeling and will can develop further: we have to start looking for a relationship to the world.

This freeing of the astral forces manifests clearly in the strength of the feelings experienced by the adolescent: joy and sorrow, hatred and love, desire, sympathy and antipathy, but also loneliness, inner pain and consciousness of mortality – all of these are intensely felt.

As our physical body is the carrier of the life body, so is the soul body the carrier of our fourth member, our spirit or I.

The I

Just like us, but unlike plants, animals also have astral bodies. But as human beings we are not limited to reflex reactions, such as is the case with animals. As human beings we are able to make our inner feelings conscious and think about them. We are able to say: 'I feel sadness,' or 'I feel hunger.' But we are capable of setting this feeling aside and, out of free will, declining to react to it. When I see something to eat and I am hungry, I can also leave it alone. This unique capacity is a complex of forces in its own right: the human I.

The I is called by different names. Aristotle (384–322 BC) spoke of the entelechy. Our word 'intelligence' is derived from it (via Latin *intelligentia*). This Greek word means: 'having the goal in itself.' The I is also indicated with the word individual, which means indivisible. The I manifests in the signature, the fingerprint, the manner of movement and the unique biography of every human being.

Our everyday I is a reflection of our higher I which does not descend at birth, but remains in the spiritual world. Because human beings have an I they are spiritual beings:

> The Holy Spirit whom the Father will send in my name, will teach you all things.
> – John 14:26

The I is our eternal, immortal, spiritual core, in which our individuality, our personality manifests itself, and to whom only we ourselves can in freedom say 'I'. Around our twentieth year our true personality is born; the I can then manifest itself and take a standpoint. We can then autonomously begin with our life tasks.

Within the limitations of their field of consciousness human beings may be alone, but also lonely. In itself, this is an extraordinary thing. We possess a form of consciousness that gives us freedom to deny the existence of what we cannot perceive through the senses. We can even deny the existence of our own creator. It is in fact a unique situation in the cosmos, where everything is interconnected, a totality, you could say the archetype of sociality. The divine has not cut us loose, but has given us freedom of choice.

On earth we can only perceive the spirit of human beings, their I-being, as a shadow, namely in their work, their deeds, their morality. In what we do we can bring something of our higher I to expression. Thus there is real meaning in the expression 'I am doing this in the spirit of ...'

> As long as the spirit is active in a physical body, it cannot work in its true form as spirit, but can only shine through the veil of physical existence, so to speak. In reality, our human thought life belongs to the spiritual world, but as it appears within our physical existence its true form is veiled. We might also say that the thought activity of physical human beings is

a shadowy image, a reflection, of the true spiritual being to
which it belongs.
– *Steiner,* Theosophy, *p. 132*

The true essence of the human being, the I-being, decides in freedom
to incarnate time and again on earth. It decides for itself, in collaboration
with other spiritual entities, what it wants to learn on earth and it makes
what could be called a life plan.

The body is the end of the road God travelled.
– *Friedrich Oetinger*

May the being of the universe
Breathe into you
The light of blessing and maturity,
The fulfilment of wholeness and balance.
– *a blessing from the Dead Sea scrolls*

In a normal state the body forms a unity with the vital forces (the life
body), while the I is enveloped in the soul forces (the soul body) with
which it also forms a unity. Both of these, the unity of physical and life
bodies and the unity of the I and soul body, move rhythmically into
and out of each other: into each other with every in-breath, out of each
other with every out-breath; into each other by day, out of each other
during sleep. However, at death, the life body leaves the physical body
and connects with the unity of the I and soul body.

In this light it is understandable that sleep is called the brother of
death; they are closely related. Birth and death may also be viewed as
in-breathing and out-breathing. As a spiritual entity, we begin to enter
the body, as it is being formed, at the time of conception, and at birth
this body, which is then 'inhabited,' appears in the world as a separate
entity and begins to breathe physically. In a breathing rhythm of day
and night and during the first half of our life, we connect more and

more with our body, whereas in the second half we gradually draw back from it again.

At night, therefore, we briefly reach back into the world from where we came, while remaining connected with the body; when we die we leave the body together with the life forces.

At death

At death the body decomposes. What it had built up goes back to its origin; the I lets the physical body go into burial or cremation, so that it dissolves into the earth or into fire. The ether body dissolves after a few days into the world ether; the astral body initially surrounds the I in the spiritual world. After a longer time it dissolves into the astral world. The I, as spiritual element, is not lost but continues its existence in the spiritual world from where it returns in a subsequent incarnation into a new physical body with new ether and astral bodies.

Immediately after death it can be clearly observed that the life body has not yet fully left the physical body and is still tenuously connected with the physical body. It seems as though the person is still breathing, as if they could still open their eyes for a moment; they may still look so alive. But within a few days the life forces gradually leave the physical body; death is then a reality also for bystanders.

In their soul the dead enter on a path that slowly but surely leads to rest. Everything connected with earthly life and living in the soul gradually comes to rest for them. That is what is meant by the well-known saying 'Rest in peace.' But the condition of the dead is not only one of rest; there is also activity. The spirit enters the spiritual world, and therefore the world of light. It is a world for which we can prepare ourselves during life. As survivors we can pray for light and rest for the soul, and ask Christ to lead it in the spiritual world.

Death is something that most distinctly has two totally different aspects. Regarded here from the physical world it certainly has many sad aspects, many painful sides. However, we really see death only from the one side; after our death we see it from the other. It is then the most satisfying and most perfect occurrence that we can possibly experience, for there it is a living fact.

– *Steiner*, Spiritual Life Now and after Death, *Nov 16, 1915, p. 9*

Whereas death proves – also in our feelings, our experience – how fragile and transitory human physical life is, from the vantage point of the spiritual world death is the sure proof that the spirit, now and always, triumphs over everything unspiritual, that the spirit, now and always, is alive and imperishable, inexhaustible life. It is sure proof that there really is no death, that death is but appearance, maya. This is also the big difference between the life from death to a new birth on the one hand, and life here on earth from birth to death on the other.

3

THE 'UNKNOWN' HOUR OF DEATH

We are not human beings who have a
spiritual experience. We are spiritual
beings who have a human experience.

Teilhard de Chardin

The Gardener and Death

A Persian nobleman:
This morning my gardener runs, white from fear,
Into my house: 'Lord, one moment, please!
Out in the rose garden I pruned shoot after shoot,
When I looked about. There stood Death.
I took fright and hurried along the other side,
But I just saw his threatening hand.
Master, your horse, let me go right away,
And I will reach Isfahan before evening.'

By afternoon – he had long since hurried off –
In the cedar park I met Death.
'Why,' I asked him, for he waited in silence,
'Did you this morning threaten my servant?'
With a smile he replied: 'No threat it was
From which your gardener fled. I was surprised,
When this morning I found him quietly at work
For I have to meet him tonight in Isfahan.'
– *from Eijck,* Herwaarts

This poem expresses the view that where we leave the earth is not an arbitrary place. In cases of sudden death, it often turns out that the one who died, or people in their circle, had had forebodings. Is sudden death then really unexpected?

I remember how busy we were with the cleaning of our future home. I was cleaning the windows when an upper window came loose and fell on my head. I was scared stiff and could only scream: 'I don't want to live here. Something horrible is going to happen here.' A year and a half later my husband suddenly died of a heart attack.

Many people ask me: 'Is the moment of death pre-ordained?' When I look back with my clients on a sudden death, we always find events and indications suggesting that what seemed sudden was perhaps not quite so. In cases of sudden death many people who are going to die do things out of another kind of knowing.

What were the last conversations about? Did the person who died finish certain things or make any arrangements? Were any conflicts resolved? An inner urge to do this may rise up from the then still unconscious knowledge of the approaching end of life.

> The day before Mother died in her sleep, completely
> unexpectedly, she told us that she had met many people in town
> whom she had not seen for a long time. And then she said:
> 'Tomorrow I am going to sleep very late.' She had never said this
> before and had also never done it.
> – *Greet*

> A young man I knew well was 22 years old. The evening before
> his death he was in a remarkably happy mood and listened for
> the umpteenth time to a song that had been a favourite of his for
> years. Its title was: 'After 22 years in this life I am making the last
> will of my youth,' and he had worn the record thin.
>   The next day on his way to work he was rammed by a truck
> and died right there from his injuries. – *Joyce*

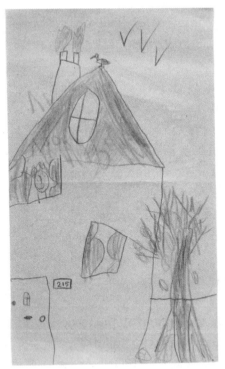 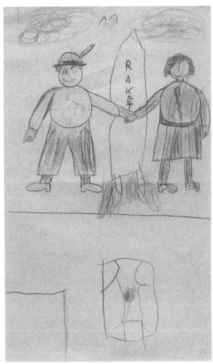

Eric was seven years old when after an illness of only a few days he suddenly died. Eric was a cheerful, spontaneous child. Shortly before he fell ill he made a drawing of a rocket being launched, fire spouting out, and mom and dad standing happily next to it. On the back he drew their house; dad had to put the house number on it. His older brother (age fourteen) is looking out of a window. This boy had a very difficult time with the sudden death of his little brother.

In the case of a fatal accident it may be important to tell the person who just died what happened, and where they find themselves now. This need not always be done aloud, it depends on what the situation allows. You can also do it with intensity in your mind.

The shock of sudden death may cause a certain black-out in the dead person. What I mean is that the observation of the situation in which the person was just before they died is more recognisable and real for them than their condition after death. You are not suddenly in another place, but you function differently in your spiritual body.

There are clairvoyants who tell us that they have seen how, for instance, in a disaster the ones who had just died tried to help the victims who were still alive. They were not yet conscious of their own situation. Bystanders can help them. The story of the 22 year old continues:

> I was the first one there. Very faintly I could still feel the last heartbeat in his neck, but he must have been killed instantly. He was lying face down by the side of the road. I sat down beside him because I did not want him to be lying there alone. Soon other people were standing around us, some five or six feet away. A doctor arrived, the police, people from the neighbourhood, and an ambulance with two paramedics. They were talking because in such a moment all kinds of things have to be organised. People wondered why it took so long before someone could give permission to move the young man to the hospital, and then it happened.
>
> I had not felt good with all the talking and all the to-do back and forth so close to the man who had just died. There had to be quiet, but how? Then it was as if an invisible tent was erected over the two of us. In that tent was quiet, peace and joy. The peculiar thing was that I could step out of that tent when someone wanted to know something or talk to me. After that I stepped into it again and found the same quiet, peace and joy. It was an extraordinary mood, a mood I had never felt before. I wonder sometimes who set up that tent over us.
> – Joyce

Sometimes just before a person is going to die, someone close to them has a sudden presentiment or a dream, or is terribly worried for no apparent reason.

> Almost five years ago I bought your book about mourning and accompanying mourning people. The reason was the death of my younger brother (then 39) in a tragic accident in the mountains. After he had fallen and died I had a visit from him

on the second night. I knew then already that he had died in
an accident. That night I was lying in bed; the world was still.
At first I was frightened by a presence and didn't dare come
out of bed, as if there were a crocodile under my bed. After
'something' came to me there was a feeling that said to me:
'Don't be afraid, your brother Gus is here.' That gave me a very
special feeling, still apprehensive, but only slightly. I started
walking through the house and – although scared and not
knowing quite what to do – I tried to talk with him.

A few weeks before his passing I had a dream about someone
who went through a black hole. In the morning I thought that
my mother was going to die. I was afraid of this dream.
– *Carolien*

Sometimes there are encounters with certain people shortly before
death, as if some contacts are intuitively initiated, or we simply run into
them.

In the 1990s I dreamed that I was lying on an operating table
with an IV in my left hand. I woke up with a very unpleasant
premonition, but I couldn't place it. That day as I was cycling to
school with my children, we met a pastor we knew and greeted
him. I went on and the premonition disappeared. Next day we
heard that the pastor had suddenly died in the afternoon of the
day we had seen him. He had been taken to a hospital and had
died on the operating table with an IV in his left hand.
– *Monique*

No, sudden is not so sudden. After the fact, such indications can be
of great comfort; they highlight a real feeling that our existence is part
of a larger life plan.

When it is not yet time

But we may also get a warning when it is not yet our time to die. Professor Eisen, who had emigrated from Sweden to America wrote to a student friend of his many years later about a remarkable event that happened to him during his student days.

> Suspecting nothing, I opened the door of my room and there, God preserve me, I saw myself lying on the bed. That I was startled is a mild way of putting it. Immediately I shut the door and remained standing outside. No, I must be seeing things. Gently I eased the door open a crack and peeped in. There I saw myself still lying on my back, motionless as if dead. I managed to shut the door again and ran into the street. Not far away lived a friend and I knocked at his door. Somewhat sleepily he opened up. I stammered some excuse which I had invented on the way, and was allowed to spend the night there on a divan. But I got no sleep that night.
>
> Next morning with the sun shining in through the window, my friend awake and his landlady bringing in the coffee, my courage and cheerfulness returned. I began to laugh out loud.
>
> 'I dare say you will want to ask what was the matter with me last night when I came rushing along half crazy,' I said.
>
> Oh, yes he would like to know. Then I told him what I had seen through the crack of my door.
>
> After some humorous comments, we decided to go and see whether I was still lying in the bed with my nose in the air. But when we opened the door, our laughter died. At the foot of the bed there had stood a tall tiled stove which we called a Swedish stove. In the night it had fallen down and had completely crushed the bed.
>
> – *from Lindholm,* Encounters with Angels, *pp. 48f*

The 'right' moment

Tolstoy described death as an unforeseen guest who appears at an equally unforeseen hour. He did view that hour as ordained from on high. As regards this view, much has changed in recent years. People used to say: 'ordained from on high' because they did not view death as chance or as something arbitrary. They believed in the knowledge and assistance of the spiritual world. They saw the course of human life as a wide arc rounding itself from birth to death in a way comparable with the dynamic of the course of the sun from morning to evening.

These days it looks as though people increasingly want to take death into their own hands, want to determine the timing themselves and carry the responsibility for it. Perhaps it is therefore good to approach the moment of death not only from the physical point of view, but to investigate it also out of the meaning of our life's destiny, which we have perhaps chosen ourselves before birth. The moment of 'sunset,' our death, might be important in the light of our sojourn on earth and what we have to develop here.

We conclude this chapter with a fairytale about the king who did not want to die.

Once upon a time there was a king who was going to die, but he did not want to. He kept his dead mother's watch under his nightshirt, and said to himself: as long as it ticks, nothing can happen to me. It also chimed the whole and half hours, and the king listened with delight to the soft tinkling sound. And again he thought: as long as that works I will remain alive, for my mother never wanted anything evil to occur to me.

This was heard by the doctor. He was a stern man. He came to the king's bed and said, 'I have to tell you: you are going to die.'

The king started. 'I don't believe it,' he said.

'No,' said the doctor, 'and yet it is true.'

'When?' asked the king.

The doctor checked the pulse and put his head on the chest of the sick man. 'It is still ticking,' he said, 'but faintly. When the leaves are falling in the garden your time has come.'

The king looked through the window and smiled. The trees were still bare and only in the bushes could you see a little green. For spring had barely begun.

'You may go,' he said, 'and call my gardener.'

When the gardener came the king was sitting straight up in his bed and his eyes were sparkling.

'Gardener,' he said, 'I am not going to die.'

'Sire,' replied the gardener, 'we must all die some time.'

'Not I,' said the king, 'chop down the trees that lose their leaves in the autumn, and plant pines and firs and holly in their place.'

The gardener did what he was told. He chopped and planted all through the summer, for it was a large garden. But when autumn came he had finished, and not a leaf fluttered to the ground.

The king was standing in his nightshirt in front of the window when he saw Death approaching. The latter looked at the garden in surprise and shook his head. But he walked on and arrived in the room of the king.

'I have to pick you up tonight,' he said, 'and yet not a leaf has come down.'

'Strange,' said the king, 'how can that be?'

'I know how,' answered Death, 'but it won't help you. Do you see that little weeping willow there? It is completely brown already. Tonight the wind will rise and then it will be bare. Why did you not chop it down?'

'I couldn't do that,' said the king, embarrassed, 'for it stands on the grave of my mother.'

Death nodded. 'I knew that,' he said, 'it is a sweet idea and for that reason I will tell you the hour. When the church bells sound half past nine I will come and fetch you.'

Death had hardly left and the king summoned his ministers.

'Take all the bells out of the church towers and smash all the clocks in the palace to pieces. Nothing is allowed to tick or sound the hours.'

The ministers did what they were told and by evening no one knew what time it was anymore. The king was standing by the window when he saw Death coming. The old man hesitated for a moment in the garden as if he was listening for something and shook his head. But he walked on and came into the king's room.

'It is time,' he said, 'I have come to fetch you. But no bells have sounded half past nine.'

'Strange,' said the king, 'why would that be?'

'I know why,' replied Death, 'but it won't help you. Just listen.'

He raised his index finger, and at that moment the hidden watch tinkled under the nightshirt of the king.

'Why didn't you smash it too?' asked Death.

'I couldn't do that,' answered the king, 'it was the watch of my mother. When she died she gave it to me.'

Death nodded. 'I knew that,' he said, 'and it is a sweet thought. Did you love her so much?'

'More than anyone else,' replied the king, and his eyes filled with tears.

'Would you like to see her?' asked Death.

The king began to weep. 'Do not tease me,' he said, 'it is my most profound wish.'

Death nodded. 'I knew that,' he said, 'and your most profound wish will be fulfilled.'

The door opened and the king clutched his heart. There stood his own mother. She bent over him and whispered something in his ear.

'Mother,' said the king, ' I don't want to die.'

'You have died already,' she replied, 'and you wished for it yourself.'

– *Bomans*, Sprookjes van Godfried Bomans

4

DEVELOPING AWARENESS OF OUR FUTURE REALM

The visible is the revelation that
disguises the invisible.

Novalis (1722–1801)

Living under the pressure of time is like continually trying to turn away from death. But if we can accept our own transience, we can liberate ourselves from this grip. If we then mourn, perhaps we mourn not because of our death, but our mortality. The more we accept the fact of death, the closer we come to a different experience of time. We then also come closer to the one who is dying, for whom timeless experience in the spiritual world is already coming into view. After death we live in timelessness. People who have had a near-death experience discover that a state of being outside the body cannot be described in terms of time, because human language is time-bound.

If we live as a conscious act of will in every moment that presents itself, time becomes more relative, wider – we can breathe! Medieval mystics spoke of *nunc aeternam,* the eternal 'now', the moment when life passes over into the eternal.

Time in the face of death

And then our time on earth is suddenly 'up'. In the face of death we inevitably wonder about the meaning of life. I have sensed the tragedy, with profound sympathy, when a dying person wondered in deep despair: 'What was the meaning of my life? What did I live for? What is the sense of it? Did it have any essential importance? It feels so empty now all that seemed so important is falling away.'

> When Peter (age 49) was told that he had but a very short time to live, the doctor said, 'You don't have much time left; do as much as possible of what you had planned to do.' Peter's reply was: 'If I now have to start doing what I had planned, I haven't lived.'

It is a grievous experience to stand at the deathbed of someone who is full of contrition, and to hear them say how happy they would be if they could live a little longer to do the things they had always dreamed of, but had always thought that they couldn't do until they had retired.

> The highest wisdom is to do that which, when we die, we would wish to have done.
> – *Multatuli (1820–87)*

Did we too often identify with the material manifestation of our existence? Do we experience ourselves only as physical beings in a world of things? We can feel so closely identified with this that another form of existence appears as hard to conceive and not credible.

If we are conscious only of bodily existence, every belief in communications about an existence after death seems like an escape from hard reality. Death then becomes like an abstract concept that applies to someone else; the reality of an end to our own life remains far away, until we are ourselves confronted with the inevitable.

We are so often distracted by what are in fact side issues in life, imposed by today's society, that there is a danger that we only live to overcome the emptiness. This is also true for time. We complain, 'I have no time, time flies.' But old Father Time is always the same. Do we have the time, or does time have us in its grip?

Due to current views and ways of life we are, as it were, pushed into situations we don't want. And yet, it is possible to stand in life in such a way that the material does not infringe upon our inner life. To achieve this we have to develop consciousness; we have to let our conscience speak. What did we know before birth? What task did we set ourselves, what did we want to develop in our earthly life, and what were our intentions before we entered into earthly life? We are completely free in doing our homework.

Consciousness, being-conscious, means development of our immortal, eternal I which, when we leave the earth, returns to our homeland.

> If you would indeed behold the spirit of death, open your heart
> wide to the body of life. For even as the river and the sea are
> one, life and death are one.
> – *Kahlil Gibran,* The Prophet

If we take this path of schooling, and have the courage to face our mortality, our sense of values will change; we become receptive to the life wisdom that is bestowed on us when we are allowed to be with someone who is dying.

That is what those who are dying teach us. They bestow on us the awareness of what is of genuine importance. When the gate of heaven opens in the hour of death, we can experience that there are not two separate worlds, but a world that is visible to our physical eyes and an invisible one, for which we need to develop different 'eyes,' a different sense of perception.

The journey to the heavenly spheres

If I prepare myself for emigration to a distant country, I try to imagine myself in that country, in my future sphere of life. I read about it, learn the language and make arrangements well ahead of time for every aspect of my approaching departure. We also do that for vacations. Why then not for our 'emigration' to the land of spirits? For there everything is totally different.

The classic example of the transition to the spiritual world is the following anecdote that dates from the Middle Ages:

> Two monks made an agreement with each other: the first to die would try to tell the other in a dream or apparition what things are like over there. They agreed on two key words: things are either *taliter* (the same) or *aliter* (different). When one of them had died he stood at night at the foot of his brother's bed and exclaimed, *'Totaliter aliter!'* (totally different).

Learning to see, learning to listen

> In the beginning of their earthly life, human beings were embryos in the wombs of their mothers. There we received the capacities and gifts for the realities of human existence. The forces and talents we needed for this world were given to us in that limited state. In this world we need eyes; we received them already in the other world. We need ears; we received them there, ready and developed for our new existence. The forces and capacities we need here were already given to us in the world of the womb.
>
> Similarly, it is necessary that human beings prepare themselves in this world for life in the hereafter. What we need in the world of the Kingdom we need to acquire here. Just as we prepared ourselves in the world of the womb by acquiring forces we need in this domain of existence, so must the rudiments of the indispensable forces of divine existence also be acquired in this world.
>
> – Abdu'l-Bahá (1844–1921), head of the Bahai faith

In the gaze of the eyes we encounter the soul; there we behold the human being, the supra-sensible human being. You can imagine that, if there are no physical eyes in the spiritual world, we must therefore on earth already develop a different capacity of perception, one using pictures, as the quotation tells us. Arthur Zajonc described it in the following striking way:

> Vision requires far more than a functioning physical organ ... Besides an outer light and an eye, seeing requires an 'inner light,' one whose luminance complements the familiar outer light and transforms raw sensation into meaningful perception.

Anne, age 42, knew that she had but a short time left to live. She called me in the spring, her voice surprised and happy: 'Now only do I see the real beauty of budding spring; I see my garden with different eyes!' Love at last sight!

> Other than the ancient Greeks, we live with a world image that is determined by science, and all too often it discounts our own active role in observation as unimportant or imagined. And yet, even today, seeing, hearing, being human, our involvement demands our continuous active participation.
> – *Zajonc,* Catching the Light

What happens at night?

> O Night, thou well of stars,
> I bathe my body and my spirit
> In your thousand suns –
> O night, that engulfs me
> In bliss of revelation,
> Disclose to me your knowing!
> O night, thou deep, deep well.
> – *Christian Morgenstern, tr. Hofacker*

We might look at the night in the following way. During sleep we do not sink into unconsciousness, but enter the spiritual world and meet beings there to whom, in our essence, we belong. There we also find those who have preceded us in death, with whom we communicate intensively in the intuitive primal language. Becoming conscious of the importance – the vital importance – of the night, is an inseparable part of preparing for death and developing consciousness of the spiritual world.

> As long as we are awake, the soul hovers above us. But when
> we sleep, part of the soul departs to higher realms. Sometimes
> an angel reveals future events to a travelling soul. In light and
> darkness.
> – *Zohar 1:183a*

At night we reflect on the past, present and future with our angel. With no one do we have such an intimately close relationship as with our angel, the entity who accompanies us from incarnation to incarnation. Our angel sees us, he protects us, he is near us when we die. He knows the entire course of our life. He knows the intentions we formed before birth, what we strive for, what we want to develop, and gives us the corresponding homework. Knowing this, having this insight, can bestow the strength on us to recognise that suffering, illness, mishap and loneliness can also be meaningful, and that life is a path of learning. Just when we are in supreme inner or outer distress or border situations, our angel is especially close. But it is important that we consciously connect with him and appeal to him. Angel (Greek *angelos*) means messenger. The angel brings us messages; he knows things about us that we don't yet know ourselves. How often we say when someone helps us at just the right moment: 'You are an angel' or experience it as 'a gift from God'?

O angel,
You who know me as no other,

Who love me without question,
Let me be worthy of you,
Teach me to love.
Grant me insight and wisdom
To understand your hints,
To bear my destiny worthily;
In confidence in your
Helping presence
In light and darkness.
– *Renée Zeylmans*

The review

The Zohar says: 'The soul testifies by night of what it does by day.'

How can we prepare ourselves for the night? An important element is the review of the day just ended. The word indicates it: re-view, look again. Look back on the important moments of the past day, from the evening back to the moment of waking up in the morning. The effort of this backward movement is like swimming against the current; it strengthens our life body.

Why this exercise? Just as we prepare for meetings, exams, important discussions, lectures, et cetera, we can also prepare for the 'conference' with our guardian angel. Everything we prepare will be more effective. The nights are crucial for our ability to function and for our insight during waking consciousness by day. The idea is not to live through everything again in an emotional way, but that we observe ourselves as from a distance. A review might last a few minutes, sometimes a little longer. But do not devote more than fifteen minutes to it.

I often imagine a mountain village. I live in the valley and climb the mountain in the evening. From there I look at the village that I can now see in its entirety, including the way I came.

In the review you might also focus on a specific subject, for instance:

- What encounters did I have, not just with people, but also with nature, animals or in other ways?
- What did I learn that was new?
- Did I listen well?
- Was I forthcoming or holding back?
- Was I perhaps spared from something? What could have happened today?

One day I told someone to do this. After two weeks she came back enthusiastically: 'You gave me such an excellent sleeping aid! I hardly get through half of the review and I am asleep.' I left it at that, for she had suffered from sleeplessness for a long time. But the idea is that you stay with it. If you do the exercise lying down there is a good chance that you fall asleep prematurely. A friend of mine has the habit of doing the review while she walks her dog at night.

You can also divide the day in two, for instance, by reviewing the morning in the afternoon and the rest of the day before going to bed. Let the events appear one by one like a slide show. Do not judge yourself or anyone else; the events are still too fresh in your memory to view them objectively. For that you first need to sleep on them for a few nights.

'To sleep on it' – time and again I experience the truth of this knowledge of old; how the night can give us clear insight when we wake up. Insight into a problem with which we have been walking around, an answer to a question, a decision that then becomes possible. During the night human beings renew their moral impulses and strengthen their ideals. The night is certainly also pre-eminently a means of arriving at self-knowledge, perhaps at mildness and forgiveness, but most of all at the insight that 'there is more between heaven and earth.' In this way the review is also a preparation for our 'journey to the heavenly spheres.'

Elsewhere in this book I describe the panorama, the three-dimensional review in the three days after dying. Some people who have a near-death experience have a preview of this. Without judgment, but focused on morality and love, we behold the life just ended.

In order to sharpen our imagining capacity even more, we can also bring to mind from time to time what we saw in nature that day, for instance, flowers in their many colour variations. We could perhaps make a flower trip and let it live on in your soul. Who can assure us that we will see the blossoms again next year? Or autumn, with its rich colours, and the trees which, full of trust in the resurrection, are moving towards their death. What we form into an inner image we will take with us to the spiritual world. Our final shroud has no pockets for material possessions, but it does for inner riches.

Ascension

It was as if the heaven
Had silently kissed the earth
So that in teeming blossoms
She couldn't but dream of him.

The air moved over fields,
The ears wove gently along
The woods were softly rustling,
The night was starry clear.

Far did my soul
Then spread her wings,
Flew o'er the silent land
As if she flew back home.
– *Joseph von Eichendorff (1788–1857)*

Contemplation: The last review

It often happens that dying people have a need to tell their life story. Relating your life story is a last review, a rounding off of your earthly life.

Frequently I hear from bystanders: 'Let the past be the past; it is too tiring for you.' However, if we as bystanders would properly understand why a dying person wants to tell their story, we would react differently. This human being wants, in the final resonance of their earthly life, to gain insight and clarity into who they were and are! They want to express who they have been.

I have often experienced how important it may be for a dying person to have the opportunity right before their death to tell their memories of the now ending life. Then I have seen them relax!

Do we have the inner silence to offer the other the opportunity to express themselves? This is only possible if we can create a loving atmosphere, if we are truly interested in the life our fellow human being has lived. We are not asked to judge or condemn. We are asked to listen. Listening means stepping into the shoes of the other, living with them, dying with them.

Let us most of all remember that what counts is not the results achieved by the dying person in their life. A result is something final, but in the spiritual world we only know the ongoing road. What we are asked is to acknowledge the courage, the strength this person has shown, irrespective of what the result has been.

In this way we can be a companion on the last 'walk' of the dying person. I have even experienced a dying person moving her feet against the end of the bed, as if she were walking her past life path one more time.

5

WHEN PEOPLE CLOSE TO US DIE

Sorrow is a holy angel,
And by him human beings have become greater
Than by all the joys in the world.

Adalbert Stifter (1805–68)

When it is a loved one who is dying we do not speak of merely escorting or attending, but of going with them. It is an immense, sometimes exhausting, reciprocal process that ends with the one remaining behind alone, and the necessity for the one dying of leaving their loved ones behind.

Together

In the quiet of evening we went together,
A path so lovely, so still with just our names.
The fairest sounds were silver crystals,
Diamonds splashed from the waterfalls.
Golden drops fell from the trees,
Pearls that flowed through rivers.
Rubies glittered in green grass,
Emeralds floated in the bog.
Blossoms fluttered brilliantly down,
Crystals made the light so tender.
Morning came, we both knelt down,
Together we thanked the Lord for this night.
When I think of this night, it is TOGETHER.

When I think of you, I say AMEN.
– *Irene Tijo**

As a loved one you also die a little

Deep connection with another
Evokes the death of who we thought we were
And the birth of something new.
– *Neil Douglas-Klotz,* Prayers of the Cosmos

The process of living towards approaching death may take years, but also months or less. It may begin the moment we receive the message that life is going to come to an end. Before that, however, there is often a time of uncertainty. Your life is going to be governed by that uncertainty.

It is a path that we each have to go on by ourselves together with others. It encompasses gradually becoming physically more dependent, and in the very last phase finally letting go. As a loved one you 'die' a little too, as it were. Sometimes you can act, arrange things; sometimes you feel powerless. To what extent can you communicate your grief, your fear and anger to the other who is going to die? Can you burden the other with that? Can you still express what you find so hard to deal with? Maybe there are situations from the past that were never expressed but are a burden? What does it mean for you to remain behind with all the troubles, cares and grief, and to have to go on alone in your mourning without being able to share anything?

The dying person may also have trouble expressing themselves. Often it is hard to find the words to voice what is taking place in the depths of their inner world.

---

*Irene Tijo wrote this poem after a profound experience at the deathbed of the man who had been like a second father to her. When dying he took her with him a little way on his path.

Some time ago a desperate woman came to me whose husband was in the last phase of his terminal illness. Could and should she still burden him with things that had never really been expressed? There is no simple answer to such a question. Sometimes it may be good for both to create clarity. But how do you do it? Out of your emotions? Or like an accusation? Have you been able to first work it through yourself?

We had a few intense discussions about it. As it turned out, she herself was still harboring a lot of unprocessed feelings she had never talked about. If she had begun a conversation with her husband out of that situation, no real communication would have been possible. She was able to process it with me, after which she no longer felt a need to bring it up with her husband. I spoke with her a year after our sessions; she was fortunately still grateful for the way it had gone at the time.

But again, things may also go differently. Sometimes it may be necessary to indeed express yourself, also for the one who is dying. Often *how* you say things is more important than *what* you say. It can resound and stay with you for a long time.

Another person may be able to make an opening, as nurse Pauli did:

It is important to realise that someone's consciousness may be dimmed, in part by medications, with the result that it is not always possible to have a conversation anymore. I remember a bedridden man whom I was taking care of at home. He absolutely refused to discuss anything about dying, although it was due to take place rather soon, at most in a few months. His wife, however, had a great need to have a conversation, and had it with me in the hallway. But it was most painful to see how little contact there was between the two partners. I had to accept the process of the man; I waited until there might perhaps come a moment when he would be open to talk. He started to have pain, and when it was clear that morphine treatments would have to begin in a few days, I said that if he wanted to talk about anything with his wife, he had to do it now. I said the same to the wife. They did find each other and talked about many things.

When he received the morphine, he indeed soon became distant (that does not need to be so with everyone). It often happens that the patient has a different way of processing things than the family or spouse.

Consolation

The dying person also has their acute struggles. Accepting is a trial, often to the end. If you are alone or have insufficient support, questions rise. Who will stay with me? Who can handle it? With whom can I talk and cry? Who can I count on? May I appeal to them, may I burden someone else?

We must not underestimate the importance of the way in which the message that the end is near is communicated, not only for the person, but also for those close to them. For them this may make itself felt long after the death of a loved one, in the way they go through mourning.

Not so very long ago, physicians were convinced that people could not bear the message, 'You are going to die.' The resulting indirectness, however, led to misunderstandings, uncertainty and distrust. But times have changed. The general approach now is to communicate the diagnosis honestly to the patient, also when there is no hope of recovery. But unfortunately, we see all too often that doctors bring this dreaded message in straightforward terms, masked by technical jargon, within the ten minute appointment, and that they take little account of the huge consequences of this information, which is in effect like a death sentence.

Mr Kay, a client of mine whose wife had cancer, told me of their conversation with the doctor when they went together to the hospital where she was being treated.

The physician said, 'We are stopping the chemo treatment; there is no point in it anymore. There are no longer any possibilities to fight the tumour. Nothing more can be done for you.'

Numbed, we left the consulting room. So that was it; not a word or gesture of compassion from the side of the doctor – just shaking hands, dismissal, next patient! Outside we tried to comfort each other, and we made the taxi trip home in silence. Only when we were home did what we were told really sink in, and we cried together.

Once you are in the hallway or in the street and you wake up to the significance of the message in all its intensity, there is often no one to help you. Just imagine being alone right then! Maybe it is possible always to have someone present in such a situation who helps the person in question, who can perhaps answer questions, but whose first task is to bring consolation.

Things can also be different, and fortunately that also happens. The American Medical Association recommends the following:

The physician also has to console the soul. This is not at all the exclusive task of the psychiatrist. It is simply the task of every practising physician.

It seems to me to be of vital importance that the doctor not only shows understanding, but that they also make their patients conscious of the fact that the life of the suffering, dying human being does not cease to be meaningful.

Intuition

It may be important to trust your intuition. When something happens it often turns out after the fact that we had a kind of premonition of it, whether it be right or not. You may be confronted with a situation that

69

doesn't feel right, although the external circumstances do not give you any reason for that, or the other way around. Physicians and nurses undoubtedly know that feeling. Then you are alert!

Sometimes you have a feeling that you have to get in touch with someone, but you postpone it. I was visiting someone in a retirement home. Afterward I felt the need to stop by another good friend living there, but I decided to come back the next day. I came too late; that same night she suddenly died. An awful experience.

Bernadette had the courage to follow her inner voice:

> Frank, the father of my son had an alcohol problem, and I had been alone since my pregnancy. When I found out that he probably had the same autism-like disorder as my son, I took up contact with him again. That was when my son was about 12. I stayed in contact with him and did not let him go again, although he gave me sufficient reason to do so. I kept it up until the moment of his death, when our contact had become most intense.
>
> He had lung cancer that had spread to his bones. Because his general physician had not taken him seriously and had only given him painkillers for a 'broken back,' he was admitted to a hospital only three days before his death. He had crawled through his house on all fours. One of his brothers, his neighbour and I were the only ones who had seen it and were doing something about it. In the hospital they did not understand how a fifty-year-old could be in such a terminal condition before being admitted.
>
> On Friday I visited him with my son and was still able to speak with him. Saturday that was no longer possible. I arranged for a private room, called his family and stayed with him until they came. They were fobbed off by the doctor on duty who said that it could still take a long time, and they left again. I went home to catch a few hours sleep.

The next day was my birthday, but I had already told my partner that he would have to have birthday breakfast by himself. At 4:30 am I woke up and sensed that I had to go to Frank. I made tea to take with me and entered the hospital very early that Sunday morning, took the elevator and stepped into the room. It was the most free decision I have ever made. I found a total chaos in the room with frantic hospital staff at a complete loss as to what was going on. Frank was in an epic death struggle. The staff were enormously relieved that someone had come to tell them what to do.

He had 'waited' for me; and after I had sat there quietly by his side for three quarters of an hour, he died, exactly at the time of my birth. I am reminded of that every year on my birthday.

Forgiving

Forgive us our trespasses, as we forgive those who trespass against us.
– Fifth petition of the Lord's Prayer

A difficult situation may arise when during life people have not been able to forgive. Forgiving and being forgiven are crucial at the end of life. If people have not been capable of doing this, it is very painful. I witness this repeatedly. Unfortunately it happens relatively often between parents and children. It is quite critical for the one who is dying.

Young and old experience the pain and injustice that have been done to them. But when you are older you can perhaps relativise things a little more; you have acquired life wisdom and are perhaps also able to put yourself in the other's shoes. When you are going to die, you often look at things with different eyes. You see your own limitations, your missed chances. What appeared so important is actually your own feeling of being offended, and sometimes the obnoxiousness, or the senselessness of your own attitude toward the other. If you feel a deep urge to ask for forgiveness or to forgive someone who has offended you, but the other does not respond because they have not yet come to that point, that makes it difficult for the one dying. It may also happen that the dying person is not ready to forgive or settle a conflict. This too has clear consequences for the mourning process of the survivors.

Forgiving always has to do with an ability to make a sacrifice, with love, and with focusing on the strong points of the other instead of condemning the weak sides. Forgiving breaks through the chain of cause and effect, of injury and retribution, Dag Hammarskjöld wrote in his diary (*Markings,* p. 197):

> Forgiveness breaks the chain of causality because he
> who 'forgives' you – out of love – takes upon himself the
> consequences of what *you* have done. Forgiveness, therefore,
> always entails a sacrifice.
>
> The price you must pay for your own liberation through
> another's sacrifice is that you in turn must be willing to liberate
> in the same way, irrespective of the consequence to yourself.

A most impressive example of this is the following Jewish prayer written in a concentration camp during World War II:

> Let an end be made to all revenge and all talk of punishment
> and retribution. There are no standards of punishment for all
> deeds of atrocity; they fall outside all boundaries of human
> comprehension. Therefore, O God, do not weigh our suffering
> on the scale of justice, do not score our executioners' deeds
> against them and do not demand from them direct and
> personal accountability for all the horrors they committed,
> but settle it in a different manner. Credit the accounts of all
> executioners, informers and traitors and all so-called evil
> people with all the courage and soul power of the tortured ones,

their subdued behaviour, their dignity, their quiet effort, their
unquenchable hope and their brave smiles despite everything
... and all love and sacrifice ... yes, the burning love in their torn
hearts which, despite everything, remained strong and full of
trust in the human being, even when eye to eye with death
and even in the hour of death, yes, also in the hours of deepest
weakness ... All this, O God, shall count for you as forgiveness
of their misdeeds, as ransom for their atrocities, so that a
resurrection of Justice may come in your humanity. Not Evil
shall count, only Good ... And in the memories of our enemies
we, the tortured ones, will no longer be their victims, their
nightmares and terrible spectres, but rather their helpers to
be relieved from madness. Only for this we pray to you. And
also, when everything is over, that we may live as human beings
among human beings. And that then PEACE may reign on this
poor earth, peace for those who are of good will ... but also for
those others, who are of bad will.
– *from* Du hast mich heimgesucht bei Nacht

In every process of forgiveness a person of necessity has to go through
an extremely painful experience, namely a feeling of inner powerlessness.
The reason is that we have to renounce any wish of retribution or
satisfaction. We have to bow our head, particularly if we have the feeling
of being in the right. In reality it is the struggle of our lower I that reaches
up to the higher I, but it is a torment, for we don't immediately succeed.
When we finally do succeed we experience the relief that a burden has
fallen away and that we and the other have become free.

In his unfinished poem *The Mysteries*, Goethe wrote:

Within this inner storm and outer struggle
Our spirit hears a word scarce comprehended:
'The power that holds constrained all humankind
The victor o'er himself no more can bind.'

Fortunately I have also been able to witness that forgiveness and reconciliation were achieved. Such peace shines forth from a battle that was fought for a long time. It is then as though we are suffused by a glowing light, as if heaven exults in the fact that we have had the strength to let the higher I triumph over the lower I.

But forgiving is always possible, even if a personal meeting cannot happen. The one who died may ask for forgiveness in a dream. When in the spiritual world after death you review your life you begin to understand why the other did something to you that perhaps dogged you all your life, but also what you did to others. You view it in an objective karmic relationship. Naturally we then develop a great inner urge to compensate. If in such a case an interaction develops between the dead and the living, it is still possible for them to arrive at forgiveness on a higher level. I have repeatedly witnessed this in my practice.

He who truly knows God
Need not forgive his brother;
He merely needs to forgive himself
That he couldn't forgive long before.
– *Leo Tolstoy*

6

THE PERSON DYING AS
FELLOW TRAVELLER

Monique van der Zanden

The last time I met Marian was on Tuesday, October 30, 2007, a few weeks before her death. She was already sick. She was suffering from pancreatic cancer. In consultation with one of her physicians, an anthroposophic doctor, she had started with Iscador, a medication that is subcutaneously injected twice a week. It mitigates pain, supports the immune system and helps retrieve some life force. 'The home care nurses are astonished,' Marian laughed.

She and Charles, her partner, had been astonished themselves when they realised that Iscador is made from mistletoe. She told me why. Around New Year she and Charles were on vacation in the Ardennes mountain range. On New Year's Day they went for a long walk. In a meadow they found an apple tree blown down in a storm. On one of the branches grew a bunch of mistletoe. They were impressed to see the plant so close up, since it otherwise always grows so high up in the crest of a tree. They studied the little leaves and the berries closely, and took a bunch home with them. That same week Marian was sick for a few days. It was a strange kind of sickness, she had never felt that way before and didn't know what it could be. And even later they never had an explanation. Exactly nine months later Marian's cancer showed up.

That Marian recounted this memory and connected it with her illness was characteristic for her. All through her life – and also now approaching death – she experienced the spiritual world as a reality, which she worked with on earth.

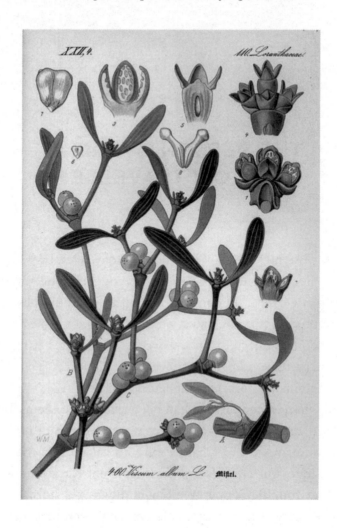

Lord, I am like to mistletoe,
Which has no root, and cannot grow
Or prosper but by that same tree
It clings about; so I be Thee.
What need I then to fear at all,
So long as I about Thee crawl?
– *Robert Herrick (1591–1674)*

The angel in every human being

I got to know Charles and Marian when I moved with my family to a home for people who had been victims of injustice or exclusion. Mutuality is the motto there: not 'I help the other' but 'We meet each other.' In that meeting people can give each other something and they learn from each other. For eleven years Charles and Marian played a key role in that organisation. Marian especially had the gift of seeing the angel in every human being, no matter how injured. Irrespective of the aversion or irritation she had to overcome in herself, she knew the art of holding back and of engaging in the battle, determined to meet the other in their deepest being. When Marian opened the door of the home she also opened her heart to the human being who was standing there.

In addition, she had a private art therapy practice, in which she worked intensively with children. Stories played a big role there; Marian liked images, spoke in images, thought in images.

In September she had major abdominal surgery, which showed that her cancer was incurable. When Marian woke up from the anaesthetic she already knew it before anyone had said anything.

'I have been up there already,' she told us later, 'and I put down my stake there. Then I came down again in confidence to walk with you all some more.'

The head nurse was dumbfounded. She confided in Marian: 'I have worked here for a long time, but I have never seen anything like it. When you came to, I saw a radiant golden light shining out of your eyes; it was unique and overwhelming.'

On the way to the threshold

Although Marian had a lot of pain she felt no anger with her abdomen. 'I carried four wonderful children in it – how can I be angry with it?' She did not experience her illness as an injustice, but did wonder what the meaning of her early death could be; for she had only just celebrated her

59th birthday. 'Perhaps after death, free from my physical body, I can give people much more than now,' she said.

She had to say goodbye, tidy her things and let go. It was a painful process in which, just as she was used to doing all her life, she surrounded herself with trusted people, choosing each for their particular skills and talents. She directed things herself and decided with which people she wanted to spend her last precious moments. The others in her very extensive circle of friends and acquaintances were kept informed by email. The cards were streaming in – many, many cards with angels on them.

In that process she also took care to heal old sores. She had conversations with people with whom she had had disagreements in the past; feelings were expressed, relationships were made whole. Marian wanted things to be cleared when she left for that other place, where new tasks awaited her.

Most of all she wished she could take her fervently beloved Charles with her a little part of the way she saw ahead of her. She grieved for him. She wanted to enable him to keep going by himself after her death by giving him a glimpse of the joyous land she sensed before her.

'I have kind of – what should I call them?' she said when I visited her that 30 October. 'Kind of death contractions – every time I am terribly afraid and sad because of everything that is happening to me, and when I succeed in letting that feeling go, rising above it, I feel myself growing very wide, wide and joyous.'

Goodbye on different levels

'We received a golden tip from a friend,' Charles told me. 'At her suggestion we started keeping a diary. Marian wrote on the left pages and I on the right. It is now a treasure for me.'

In the diary Charles and Marian addressed each other:

November 4, Marian:
[Her desk was given to someone today. She had to cancel a planned dinner with some friends, but encouraged Charles to go anyway.]
A day for crying; the tears well up and stream down. I don't want it but I can't help it. Saying goodbye hurts! With my desk seven years' work, great work, are also gone. Little plans like going out for dinner also make things harder when I don't have the strength.

I am so glad that everyone sympathises with me, cries with me or eats with me; and you ... wonderful that you can go!

Tomorrow a day for laughing?

I hope so!

November 15, Charles:
[Today a friend came to visit who accompanied Charles and Marian; she is a holistic therapist who works with energies.]
At your bed we had a nice trio today with E. It was a good conversation. There are so many people who help us so much.

November 15, Marian [reacting to that conversation]:
The day of the Mystical Marriage of Charles and Marian. I need you so much, Charles, and you are so with me! Such a rich piece in our life together, and we are doing it!

The night from November 17 to 18, was a sleepless night. Marian had terrible pain. The cancer had reached the spleen. On the 18th she began with morphine, although it was against her principles. E. reassured her: when you have so much pain that you can't think of anything else, or resolve things you still want to take care of, then it is better to take painkillers.

November 20, Marian:
I develop from earth to metal: from painful spleen to mildness –
two clenched fists of holy rage.

No old patterns, but sensing space to come to decisions,
letting go, handing over. Grateful for relief of pain and of ideas!

November 23, Charles:
Many pictures move through you, as in a film.

November 23, Marian:
It is at a little distance that I am writing this, not so direct, for
there is a lot involved in saying goodbye, and on different levels.
Time and space play roles of their own in this, very differently
from what we are used to. Perhaps I will explain it some time,
not now.

November 24, Marian [ten minutes before she died]:
There is so much left when you think you don't have anything
in your hands anymore…

Pure soul

Saturday afternoon around noon a friend brought a work of art she
had made herself: an angel. Twelve hours later, around midnight,
while walking to her bed to go to sleep, Marian suddenly died of a
cardiac arrest.

That whole evening she had been with Charles, a musician in heart
and soul. Together they listened to music by Bach, like they did every
evening during her illness. This evening she let him choose, and she
asked him about certain technical aspects of the music. She also leafed
through his professional journals, something she never used to do.

'It was as if she wanted to tell me, "Keep doing what is important for
you", said Charles. At the end of the evening he thought that she was

strangely quiet. He was the only one with her when she died. His name was her last word.

Tenderly he related how serenely she went through her illness and death process. 'Holiness radiated out from her,' he said. The origin of the word holy lies in the word whole. As a friend said: 'Marian lived death and life as an organic whole.'

Marian died at home and was laid out at home. The night before her funeral, after the three days between dying and burial that she had always considered so important, Charles had a dream.

> I went into a cellar, a system of passages. It had a little light, and in front of me was a deep, dark hole; a stairway led downward. Then I heard a call and looked to the right. I saw a long passage and at the end on the right was a shining light. And there was Marian! She came walking backward out of the light toward me. She was heavily pregnant and collapsed in front of my feet, dead. I exclaimed, 'Marian, you can't do that. You are dead!'

Charles still feels the joy of that dream. It confirmed him in his feeling that her physical body may be dead, but that she is filled to the brim with new life. He also sees the dream as a message from Marian that her path did not lead down the stairs into the dark, but that she went through a long passage to the light.

It gave him the strength at the funeral to play music for her himself. Everything was done the way Marian had wanted it: a friend painted an angel on the cover of the casket, someone else took care of the flowers, Marian and Charles's children carried the casket, there were beautiful texts and candles: 'You may laugh, dance and make music!'

When we had buried her we came together with apple turnovers! What else did we expect? Whenever a lot of work had been done Marian would make apple turnovers. Not for nothing she called them 'work turnovers.'

On November 29 Charles wrote on the memorial card:

Here on earth you were already closely connected with the
spiritual world. You, dear Marian, pure soul. How much I need
you, Marian. But full of gratitude and full of love and pride
I hand you over to the spiritual world, where our Mystical
Marriage continues for all eternity!

As long as I lived there, Marian and I did the weekly shopping for the
organisation. We always went to the farmers' market. A few days after
Marian's burial I went, as usual, to the market in my current home town.
And there she greeted me – the side of a flower stall was full of bunches
of mistletoe! They had never had those before.

Eyes full of light

On November 18 I wrote a fairytale for Charles and Marian; it was born
out of grief and from a very special inspiration when I woke up. Only in
January I heard from Charles the story of the nurse who had said, 'When
you came to, I saw a radiant golden light shining out of your eyes…'

The Magic Door

Once upon a time there were a man who made music and a lady
who told stories. They wandered from town to town, and in every
town he played music that opened the hearts of people, and then
she told a wondrous story. It was the story of the magic door.

The magic door is a golden door, and behind it shines a
golden light. Whoever sees that light immediately falls in love
with it and wants to see ever more of it. The story of the magic
door is the most beautiful story in the world.

One day the musician and the story-teller arrived at a large
house in a city, and they decided to live there for a while. The
musician played his music that opened the hearts of the people,

and the story-teller told her story of the magic door, and everyone was welcome.

Not long afterward the doorbell rang during the music. The story-teller walked to the door of the large house (which was not made of gold) and said, 'Look, this is the magic door.'

She opened it. 'Do you see the golden light?'

The people who had listened to the music and the story were surprised and looked out.

'Not really,' said one, 'I see a street full of noise and blowing paper.'

'No,' said the next one, 'I see pouring rain.'

'No,' said a third, 'I see a shivering man with dirty clothes and a hungry look in his eyes.'

'Exactly,' said the story-teller. 'His eyes are what I mean. I will teach you to look. In the eyes of that man the golden light shines.' The people looked closely, and after a long time, during which they remained quiet, they said, 'Now you mention it, I believe I see something.'

For eleven years the musician and the story-teller stayed in that large house with the magic door. They taught many people how to look. 'Don't be afraid of what you will see on the other side of the door, even though you don't know it,' they said. 'If you look carefully you will always see that beautiful golden light again.'

And that was true. More and more people were able to see it, and once you see it you fall in love with it right away. In this way the shivering, hungry, grieving, angry and desperate, troublesome and sick people on the other side of the door became like brothers and sisters.

After eleven years had passed the musician and story-teller said, 'We have to go.' And the story lady added: 'The time has come that I may go through the golden door to the golden light and become part of it.'

The people were surprised and exclaimed: 'Don't go! We can't yet do without you. Often when we open the door we only see the grey street, the angry wind, or those fussy people. Who will teach us to look?'

The musician played his most beautiful music and the story-teller smiled. She said: 'From now on you have to do it yourselves. You have learned enough. Now you just have to practise.'

But the people cried. They called, 'But we can't do without you; we love you so much, you mean so much to us!'

And a woman said softly: 'When you are gone from the large house we can still visit the musician and listen to his beautiful music. But you, story-teller, when you have gone through the golden door, we will never see you again.'

'You can see me more often than ever before,' said the story-teller with her sweetest smile. 'Remember, I become part of the golden light. Every time you open the magic door and look closely into the eyes of the person who is standing there, you can meet me.'

7

WHEN YOUNG PEOPLE DIE

During the first twenty years of our lives the life forces are stronger than the forces of destruction. Then follows another period of about twenty years when the constructive and destructive forces are in balance. From about age forty, the destructive forces become stronger than the constructive ones, with the result that the body physically begins to show age. Thus we live with death. Goethe called this principle in our life: 'Dying and becoming.'

Sometimes people die young.

How wrong and grievous to have to leave the earth when you have been there but a short time! You are in the middle of the building phase, you have your whole life in front of you, and suddenly everything is torn down.

Marina

I experienced that with my daughter-in-law, Marina; she was only 27. She had just moved in with her partner and had graduated as a teacher with the wish to be a kindergarten teacher. Then came the message that she had a brain tumour. Due to the necessary medications and radiation it became more and more difficult for her to move about, whereas she was such a cheerful person. Now she had to slow down and pull back more and more.

We were sitting at the kitchen table and she asked: 'Do you think there are also toddlers up there?'

I answered in the affirmative: 'Maybe you can mean a great deal for children who died young.'

'Then I want to be there for them!' Hope rose in her eyes, hope for the future.

Not long before her passing Marina wrote a poem in her diary that we later printed on the announcement of her death.

> When this skin has done its job
> And has for good been laid
> Under the grass, I shall,
> After years of fear and dread,
> Reenter the room which was
> The room of my life.
> – *Adriaan Roland Holst*

From her earliest youth, Marina lived at a fast pace and with intensity, a phenomenon we can witness frequently. People who die young have to get as much as possible out of life in a short time.

John

We can also see that in the story of John.

> John was, I believe, the oldest of our youth group. He was 24. Whenever he could, he was there every Friday evening. But he couldn't always manage that because John had had polio as a child. He was badly handicapped, in a wheelchair and could hardly move. He needed help for everything.
>
> But John was also the merriest of the whole group. He never stopped asking about all we had done that week and drank the information in. It was as if he had experienced it all with us and delighted in it again when we told him of it. His face then looked very youthful.
>
> John's health deteriorated, he became weaker and could no longer come to our meetings. Shortly afterwards came the

news that he had died, suffocated in his own mucus that he could not cough up.

We went to say goodbye to him. The viewing was in his home. He was no longer the merry, almost youthful John. An old man was lying there. With a shock I realised that in the 24 years of his life John had lived through an entire life of perhaps 60 or 70 years. He had done it much faster than we had, and could therefore die now.

– John's friend

We have in our world pushed our mortality to old age. The question of why comes strongly to the fore in people who die young and those around them. Questions of meaning and sense. We wrestle with thoughts like: this death cannot be meaningless; then birth would also be meaningless! Meaninglessness is deadly.

In Marina I had seen acceptance, not the wish to accept, but true acceptance. She had perspective reaching across the threshold; death for her became another form of life.

Marlene

Young people's battles may also last until the moment of dying, as it did for Marlene. At age nineteen Marlene contracted leukemia. She underwent intense radiation. When she was 25, the disease came back. She was then living together with her friend Wiard. Thanks to alternative treatments and food, her positive attitude and her will to live, she had a reasonably good life for a year and a half. But then the leukemia hit her hard so that she had to undergo the most intensive chemo treatments.

Marlene kept a diary that she shared with others on her website. I received permission to include her and Wiard's story in this book.

Early October 2004
Everything has gone very differently than expected. After a

month in the hospital – with the most difficult chemo course
I have ever had – I was going to go home for four weeks
to recuperate, before I had to undergo the next treatment.
Four weeks looked good to me, except that the day after
my discharge from the hospital I had a heart examination,
because during the chemo it had given me some problems.
The outcome of this was that I had heart problems caused by
serious damage to the pumping function of my heart, probably
due to an accumulation of certain chemicals. In my case it
involved the left chamber, the pumping function that sends
blood and oxygen to all organs.

Both my friend and I were deeply shocked by this news
and again had to process a lot. Not only did I now have a heart
problem, but the chemo could not be continued because
my heart would not be able to handle intensive chemo and
radiation. With all our positive thinking we tried to convince
ourselves that the leukemia would stay away and that we could
now fully concentrate on healing my heart.

My cardiologist does not believe that my heart can recover,
at any rate, he has never seen that. If I had not been a leukemia
patient he would have placed me on the waiting list for a heart
transplant.

All right, in the meantime we continued to look for
information about heart failure. I have been investigating
orthomolecular medicine for a while and, although I am still
very tired, retain a lot of fluid and have to cough a lot, still,
the tightness in my chest was gone in a month, so that I can
fortunately breathe freely again. I am incredibly happy with
that, for it is really awful when you have trouble breathing.

Late October
We had a wonderful week in Switzerland with the family, in
a spot where we have gone for almost twenty years. I wanted

to go at all cost, and went against the advice of the doctors. Everything went well. The family took wonderful hiking trips every day, and Wiard and I made leisurely visits to places like Interlaken, Bern, Thun and Spiez. Our food was beautifully taken care of and all we had to do was enjoy things. That wasn't hard. We laughed a lot with each other and played a lot of games together.

Back at home things got tough. All that time I had put little braids in my hair against hair loss (a good tip if you want to keep your hair as long as possible). I had already had an itch on my head, and here and there you could see a bump. I also had a rash on my stomach. When Wiard shaved my head it proved to be full of big red bumps. When I saw my doctor he immediately referred me to a dermatologist for a biopsy, for my doctor thought immediately of the leukemia. Despite all my fears, I still wanted to believe that it was some sort of skin disease, but oh, the wait for the test results was tough! I had a really hard time with it.

Two days earlier than planned we received the message: the leukemia is back. It was also in my blood. This meant that two or three weeks after the intensive chemo treatment the leukemia was already back, for that was when I began having the skin rash.

So that was it; at least that was what we were living with for a few days. Finished with the hospital, no good prospects, no physician who could help me anymore.

December 21, 2004. (Wiard writes together with Marlene)
To finish her story, she picked up the thread again and with her strong will began to work on 'getting better'. However, in order to suppress the proliferating leukemia cells she needed a low dose of chemo. Her energy was slowly broken again, and her blood count decreased rapidly. As a result she was in the hospital twice a week for blood transfusions.

Time and again she managed to crawl out of the low spots where she got stuck all the time. Time and again she astonished me and others by being with us as if nothing was happening. She thoroughly enjoyed a Flamenco performance after Christmas, and on Christmas day we were with her family in Belgium, and the day after with my brother and his partner. New Year's Eve we celebrated at home with friends; it was great!

Marlene passed away on 7 January 2005 at age 27.

Wiard:
At one point things looked as if everything was under control. The chemo continued to be effective, the leukemia was under control, the blood varied, but she still improved with the transfusions, albeit not much. Then came a time in the New Year when I saw her naked, and I had a fright. I asked her to step on the scale and wow, even though she was already ten kilograms [20 lb] under her normal weight, she had lost another three [6 lb].

On Monday January 3, she had diarrhea. Nothing else. A day later her temperature rose slowly. By evening it rose faster and reached 40.3°C [104.5°F]. I got antibiotics for her and they worked, but not for long. Fever suppressants and antibiotics were hardly able to handle the fever.

January 6, 2005
The day ended with tightness in the chest so that breathing became more difficult and the pain in her back got worse. She could not find a position in which she could comfortably lie without pain. The night was long, and the next day her shortness of breath became worse, as did the pain. At one moment she literally said: 'I have had enough.' And yet she did

not want to admit that things were going badly. She was simply planning to get better. Then when the doctor came and gave her a morphine injection to decrease her difficulty breathing and take away as much as possible of the pain, her last words were: 'I am going to sleep.' She was then still conscious for twenty minutes, during which I gave her a little water now and then to moisten her mouth.

Soon after, she lost consciousness, breathed in, and stopped breathing. It took a short while before she breathed out again and died in my arms… For me an incredibly difficult moment and one of unbelievable pain and grief. I was alone, and in that condition gave expression to my deep, primal emotions that then came to the surface. I screamed as hard as I could, and I cried my heart out.

For three days Marlene stayed with me at home, lying in a bed in the living room. I am glad to have done this. It was good to say goodbye to her in this way. We had a constant stream of visitors with whom I could share my grief, people who gave me much support. Thank you all!

On Wednesday 12 January we buried her.

From Wiard's diary, after Marlene's passing:

October 28, 2005
Darling, I miss you!
I long for the moment of my passing,
the moment when our souls will meet in light and love.

November 2, 2005
I don't find it hard to see the meaning of life;
I find it hard to feel like living again.

In December 2005 Wiard met his Marlene again in a dream:

Early this year, my darling died of leukemia. For five years we were together. I have a lot of grief, and these past few weeks this became again a suffocating grief. Thus goes my mourning, with ups and downs. My grief veils my soul in the spiritual world; this is something I am conscious of. Sometimes I can set this grief aside and feel gladness for her birth into the spiritual world.

Two nights ago I had an experience I have never had before. I had an incoherent dream that I could remember when I woke up. This is unusual, because normally I don't remember my dreams. In this dream she suddenly stood next to me and radiated happiness and love. I was also glad for this reunion; it was really a great surprise. We immediately took each other in our arms, and I felt how a very intense feeling of love came over me. It was such an intense feeling, so real, that I knew without a doubt that this was Marlene, this was the soul of Marlene who said to me here: 'I love you.' Full of this love, I woke up sobbing from this dream. I had to cry my heart out. I am very grateful and have expressed this in the past few days: thank you so much, my darling, for your visit, thank you for your love.

Wiard experienced how until age 35 people still have strong up-building forces in them, forces they brought with them at birth from the spiritual world. When they die young, they have not yet completely used them up. People who die young take these forces with them again when they 'go home.' That which they were not able to achieve on earth they can bestow on earthly human beings.

8

EXPERIENCES IN A CHILDREN'S HOSPITAL

Patricia de Vos

When a child is dying, you can only become very still. How do you accompany a child to the end of their short life on earth? Patricia de Vos interviewed with great care and love several parents who lost a child; she also spoke with doctors and nurses who accompanied the young patients and their families in this always heart-rending journey.

What do you meet on this journey through a land of pain? What do you do? What don't you do? What is important?

In the pediatric haemato-oncology department at the hospital where I work, children from birth up to the age of sixteen are admitted who have cancer, serious blood diseases or immunity disorders. Fortunately most of them are cured, but inevitably death, and accompanying children to their death, are part of the work.

In these contributions, after the death of their child, parents take the reader along on a journey which one hopes that no one ever has to make with their own child. At the same time, however, they are all silent witnesses of courage and inner strength, of unconditional love between parents and their child.

Professionals also had a chance to contribute from their experiences. When a cure is no longer possible they each handle that in their own personal manner.

Bad news

How as a parent do you tell your child that they are going to die?

> When Arco still wanted to ride his bike, I said to him: 'You are
> not strong enough for that.' He replied: 'But when I am well
> again, then I can do it!' I then told him that he would not be
> well again. He asked me: 'Then what is going to happen to me?'
> While I held him close to me I said to him: 'Your little
> body remains behind, and you come back home with us.' I did
> not want to tell him that he would be cremated, so as not to
> scare him. He was reassured and never came back to it until
> his death. But it was the most difficult thing I have ever had to
> do in my life.
> *– Arco's mother*

As physician you face the task of having to bring bad news.

> With certain children I quickly have a kind of uneasy feeling,
> and then there is the niggling thought that one day I will have
> to give the bad news or have a palliative conversation. And yes,
> this has an influence on the relationship with the child and the
> family. In most cases I strive for an equilibrium between giving
> hope and not raising expectations. But when that uneasiness is
> there I will perhaps give a little less hope.
> Bad news conversations with the children themselves,
> especially the older ones, the adolescents, are difficult. I feel
> that it is our task and not that of the parents to tell them that
> there is nothing more we can do. I will tell the parents, 'If they
> start shooting, let them shoot the messenger.' But after a death
> I always feel terrible.
> On the one hand, people want figures; on the other hand,
> sometimes we can also hide behind figures, statistics and theories.
> There may be questions of what can still be done, or what

is still possible in the way of palliative care. In other words, concrete questions with concrete answers.

Parents sometimes ask me: 'What if nothing works anymore? Can we get any help?' If the future is hopeless it is not so hard for me to accept that a child is dying; also, talking about death is not so difficult for me. However, we also witness how some people reach their limits; pain medication is then very important. Continuing a treatment against our better judgment is something I do not agree with. And sometimes you have to let yourself be guided by the child. As physician you have to be able to listen carefully to what the child still wants.

Death is never nice. We must not tell parents that we can always ensure that death will occur serenely, without pain, bleeding or anxiety. But even if the child dies serenely and beautifully, it is still a tearing away of a child, a person, a loved one out of our life. That hurts! It may not always be unexpected, but it is always unpleasant.

The story of Luke

Luke was barely two years old when he died of a brain tumour. Here is the story of his parents.

After ten months of treatments, surgery, chemotherapy and radiation followed a first moment of respite. We are in a convalescence home and are almost embarrassed by the care and attention we are receiving. And our Luke, for the first time in almost a year, may do again what all children do: play and romp together.

We have a wonderful Christmas, until Luke tires visibly and shows the first signs of pain. Our gut feeling is not good. Something in our body sounds the alarm. The doctor reassures us, and we have a period – the only period in the whole process – when we feel a lack of understanding. Luke goes from examination to examination, and every time there is 'good' news: they didn't find anything. No one seems to understand how this 'good' news, as we experience it, always brings the drama closer. These are days between hope and despair.

One Sunday Luke has an urgent MRI scan. Finally! After a short wait, we get the result: the cancer has not come back. We breathe a sigh of relief. But Luke is more poorly all the time and when touched, clearly signals that it hurts.

In the meantime it seems as if the tension around the whole process has little impact on our two daughters; it seems to pass them by. Is that because of all the Christmas excitement, or are they sparing us? Sometimes we think the latter was then already happening.

On Tuesday January 6 again an MRI. We wait for the result. The doctor comes in; we can tell from her demeanour that something is coming. 'It is not at all good. We can see on the scans that the tumor has metastasised to the back.' We hardly hear the rest. We look at each other and wait for the verdict.

'What are his chances? And what now?' we ask.

'We don't think we can do anything anymore,' says the doctor.

A deadly moment in our life, very difficult to describe. Everything almost literally becomes cold, breath is cut off, we look at each other in despair. The doctor takes a long time to help us through the first horror. She stays with us and asks whether we want to see a psychologist. We do want that, but do we actually still know what we want? We hold on to each other, and can only stammer a bit. We are losing him; it can't be true, we are dreaming. It can't be. We may have said that a hundred times to each other.

Then come the telephone calls to close family and friends.

Two weeks of visits that are all meant to be supportive but also take a lot of our time. Luke is sitting there and watches television. He is little child of two; does he have any idea of what is happening?

Then we had to tell the bad news to Luke's two sisters. We want to break it gently to them, but as soon as we come in there is no need to say anything anymore. The children know right away what the story is and we all embrace each other. There is a lot of crying, few words. No, it had not passed them by at all, on the contrary.

Luke's life expectancy is now two months; in the end it turns out to be 14 days.

On Monday January 11 we have an appointment with the head of the children's cancer department of the hospital. He takes more than an hour to show us that the cancer is incurable. He gives us a very difficult message in a very human way. We could still choose for very intensive chemotherapy, but the chance that this will save his life is one percent. And the chance that his life will then be worthwhile is also one percent. One percent of one percent... And the certainty that it would entail great suffering is very great. It is tough indeed, but it helps us to decide on the path of palliative care.

We join a hospice organisation for children. We are told that in the beginning they will visit very often, but will not push themselves on us.

Luke's struggle with death is not nice. His condition deteriorates so quickly, and there are great difficulties to control the pain. Every day is a battle. In several books we read that many things are often still possible to do with a dying child, but in our case, almost nothing turns out to be possible. Any break or day trip we had hoped to make proves to be impossible because of the cancer.

We can't get Luke's pain under control. Until about five

days before his death he is conscious, albeit less and less so. When he is awake he is very frustrated and demands that we constantly sit where he wants us to sit, and stay there, sometimes for a long time. He is also very irritated with the nurses as well as with his sisters who are playing and romping around before his eyes. A few weeks earlier he could do that too, but now no longer. We indulge every wish, every whim, every show of anger; there is no need any more for parental control.

As the cancer strikes deeper Luke has periods of terrible screaming alternating with total exhaustion, in the arms of his mother. We increase the dosage of the pain medication, but it does not help. Finally he gets a painkiller that keeps him asleep most of the time. As soon as he shows signs of unrest, he receives another dose, and that works. He hardly reacts to us those last few days until a remarkable, lucid phase the evening before his last day. Then he drinks a little and obviously reacts to us. For the last time. Those last days he sleeps between us so that, should he quietly pass away, he would at least not be alone in his bed.

On 20 January we wake up, and just as on the first day, it is Mom who sees that something has changed. On the day of Luke's birth she had said that she had a strange feeling, as if she expected that something would go wrong with this child. Now she saw that this was indeed going to happen.

The last days of Luke's life were a matter of survival for us. Fortunately we had much help from a network of family and friends. We are most grateful for their support. Around one o'clock, in the arms of his mother and with dad and the sisters around him, Luke quietly leaves us. No panic, no screaming, but in silence and in the midst of the people he had always wanted around him. A beautiful way of dying, but otherwise really hard to digest.

Being and remaining present:
a psychologist's viewpoint

A psychologist follows the family during the entire treatment phase, and builds a relationship of trust with the child and the family. Accompanying a person means learning, searching.

The fear of death, of the unknown – perhaps we are born with it. We feel uncertain in it. We become aware of great powerlessness, and as psychologists we have to learn how to deal with that, because we can offer nothing concrete. The important thing is to be and remain present. No running away despite sitting in darkness, despite the fact that there are no signposts in or out.

Actually, the parents have taught me a great deal. They took me with them into this world of dying children. Parents' reactions like, 'You don't need to say anything; just be present, that is enough,' have given me courage. In my view it is our task to recognise and to connect with the whole family. And at the same time we have to stay somewhat in the background.

What we experience in our work is something we can't relate to many people without appearing to feel like a victim, or to appeal for compassion. Do we then have to be 'hard' to be able to do this? No, certainly not, on the contrary, I feel myself becoming ever more vulnerable. Maybe it is because of growing older, or because of my own children who are growing up, that I have become better able to identify with the parents and really live in their situation. But saying things like 'I understand you,' or giving advice, are like traps – they only provoke irritation.

With teenagers you have a double pain, that of the parents and that of the young person who really wants to live but isn't given the chance. That is something you bring home with you. As parents you go through hell, but also as caregiver you go through a mourning process. But that goes unrecognised; you have to do it completely by yourself.

I carry all the children who have died with me, including in my life outside the hospital. At our wedding, and at the baptism of our children I felt the need, when choosing the Bible texts, to make a connection with those who will never have this opportunity. You also learn to relativise in your own life.

Respect and accept: nurses in oncology

Our department has a whole crew of nurses who commit themselves day after day to the patients and their families. Care in all its multiple aspects forms the golden thread in their work. It does not leave them unmoved when a child is seriously ill or is incurable.

> To work in such a place you have to be special; this holds
> true for everyone, doctors, nurses, yes, also the cleaning crew.
> Throughout the treatment of my daughter I viewed them a
> little like family. They took care of my daughter the way we
> did at home. Everyone was friendly and did what they could
> to support us in this difficult time. You didn't realise what they
> all did for you in the moment. It was often the little things for
> us parents that were so important. Their sensing of the little
> details made us always feel important.
> – *A parent*

Some parents have accepted the facts; others are not yet able to believe it. With the latter it is more difficult to send them home with confidence in their heart.

When a doctor unexpectedly starts speaking about palliative care, reality suddenly forces itself on the parents; that may be hard to bear. However, a brief illness, a sudden death, or little time between palliative care and death may be just as difficult.

Some things make it more difficult or easier, for instance: are you strong within yourself, is there acceptance by the family? If the time the child was treated in the hospital was very long I sometimes experience the death as a deliverance for the child. If there is acceptance, it is easier to see the good things – the child fought with all their strength, and everything was done that could be done.

As caregiver you have to respect and accept the reactions of parents when their child dies, or their decisions as to the place where this happens, whether or not this makes things easier or more difficult for you.

When a child dies in the hospital it is important that the caregiver is familiar to the family. After the death the room has to be vacated... But you have to give people time... Let them do it themselves, or ask them if you can help.

Colleagues are important; you can briefly unburden yourself with them; their strength helps you when you enter the room of the dying child.

Among nurses and other caregivers there are great differences in how they feel about attending the funeral of a child. Personally, I do that, both for the parents and for myself. On the other hand though, as caregiver you do have the right to set a boundary, to say: 'I can't do that.'

The story of Debbie

One day Debbie, a teenager, was told that she could not be cured. Debbie, her parents and younger brother – each in their own way – had to wrestle with overwhelming grief, feelings of powerlessness, anxiety and uncertainty. But there were also good moments, for Debbie tried to get everything out of her 'being young,' and the parents gave her all their time and love, and tried to make the best of the most ordinary things. Here are the words of her father and then of her mother.

> It was a terrible moment when my wife and I heard that she could not be cured. All we could do was to give her all our

attention. The home carers from the hospice were so good –
their people also gave attention to our son.

Debbie never talked directly with me about the fact that
she was going to die, but she knew it. One day we were talking
about going to the beach for a few months. Debbie said then,
'Yes, but with the three of you, Mom. Dad and Jonas.'

She knew very well that she would not be there anymore...

Debbie's first words after the verdict: 'I agreed to this treatment
to please you, but as far as I am concerned, I don't need it
anymore.' Debbie continued to fight so as not to disappoint us,
but for her the battle was over.

When we came home she asked us to call her best friend.
She needed to be comforted. Apparently her father and I were
too upset to give her real consolation. For Debbie there were
two choices: waiting for death or enjoying life as much as
possible. Fortunately she chose the latter and the cancer did
not prevent her from enjoying things and gaining experiences
in the time that remained to her. She went out with friends
as much as she could. Just as with every healthy adolescent,
parents did not fit into this picture.

I never made a fuss about this. I never begrudged her any
moment of pleasure. On the contrary, she was happy, and I was
too. She felt free and happy, and I was happy because she was. I
had to share her with many people, and I was happy to do that.
The only thing that mattered was what she would enjoy, and I
absolutely did not want to keep her away from that. But every
time she went out I was anxious. Only when she came home
was I at ease again. Strange, in a way – you know that your child
is going to die, but the anxieties don't go away.

Sometimes I had the impression that Debbie felt guilty that
she went out and we stayed at home. She often urged us also to
go out. Once she said to me that it would be all right with her

if I went back to work; I could stay at home when she would not be able to get out of bed anymore. I told her then that it was my greatest task to be at home with her, and that this was absolutely necessary for me to be able to live with myself later.

The last day we were at the beach she found a gift for each of us. She sensed that she would not last much longer. Goodbye presents? Never-forget-me presents?

When Debbie could no longer get up the stairs we put her bed downstairs, and I emptied a cabinet to put her things in it. Among her things was a pair of jeans that were completely frayed at the bottom. I asked if she still needed those, to which she replied yes. I did not want to dash her hopes; I was also hoping for a miracle.

We never really talked about death. My effort to arrange for her to talk to a psychologist was turned down by Debbie. She did not want to talk with me about death or her feelings about it. She promised to do this later perhaps, but in writing. I had to respect her wish. Unfortunately she never put anything on paper. Maybe she thought this was better, and perhaps she was right. Her true thoughts might well have made us even unhappier.

During Debbie's terminal period hours and days all flowed into each other. We had lost all awareness of time. Every morning I rose early. Every morning I cried my heart out so I could then be cheerful during the day and make Debbie happy. I did not want to show her my grief, so I wouldn't make her sad. One time I tried to have a conversation about that with her. I told her that I often cried and asked her if she did too. 'Yes,' she said, 'in my bed,' and she turned her back to me and went upstairs, probably with tears in her eyes. Evidently, she did what I did: she hid her grief from me. It is darned difficult to show each other your grief when you are so close.

When Debbie could no longer get out of her bed, she totally changed. Texts and emails from friends remained unread.

She slept a lot and watched television. She used to love books, but she suddenly stopped reading them. Interest in life melted away like snow in the sun. Her friends were no longer her first concern. We, her parents, became the most important people for her.

I no longer slept in my bed but in a chair, to watch over her and help her in case of problems. Debbie praised me for that without many words, but I knew and sensed her love for me. One day she said to me: 'Mom, you are always there when I need you. Wouldn't every mother do that for her child?' She wanted my confirmation that this was simply part of what a mother does. Nothing abnormal. Feelings of guilt?

In her last hours she wanted me close to her; I couldn't leave the room anymore. I suggested that I get into bed with her and hold her in my arms, but she could not tolerate my body against hers. I did have to hold her hand. I told her that I loved her very much and that I would always think of her as a good, intelligent, courageous girl, a daughter to be proud of. She smiled and I knew that she could now die with a clear conscience.

The last words she spoke to me were: 'It isn't fair, Mom.' My girl wanted to stay alive; she loved life. In a way it was comforting that evidently we had not done so badly with her, but I will never, never forget those words.

Looking back, I know we did our best. At any rate, I am very glad that Debbie was able to be at home in her terminal period, that she was able to die at home, and that I was able to take care of her. For me this was a great consolation, and I think that it was for Debbie the greatest gift we have ever been able to give her. Yes, Debbie, I have always been proud of you, even when you were ill, even when you had to use a wheelchair. Everywhere I went with you I said to myself: 'Look, people, this is my daughter, my child. Look how courageous she is, bearing her martyrdom without complaint.'

Debbie, now I realise how our relationship subtly changed when you fell ill – a relationship of trust between the two of us that grew and grew until you died. I am so happy that you let us feel in the last weeks of your life that we, as parents, came first for you, that you needed us.

Remarks from a hospice nurse

Children often give signals, verbally or non-verbally, that they are aware of the fact that they are going to die.

A very ill toddler told his parents on Christmas Eve to set the table with their pretty Christmas things. The parents were so sad that they didn't feel like celebrating Christmas. But they did it for their little son; it was his last Christmas.

Some children seem to wait for their parents' presence before they die.

It used to be taboo to talk about death; parents did not do that with the dying child or the other children. Sometimes, however, it turned out, perhaps through a diary or similar, that the dying child or the brothers and sisters knew perfectly well that death was approaching.

II

CARE FOR THE DYING

Do not fear, I am the LORD your God.
When you pass through the
waters, I will be with you;
and when you pass through the rivers,
they will not sweep over you.
When you walk through the fire,
you will not be burned...
Do not be afraid, for I am with you.

Isaiah 43:1–5

9

THE SENSES OF THE ONE DYING

During our growth phase, as human beings we have to connect with the earth and our bodies through our senses, whereas a dying person has to learn the opposite, namely to let go of the earth and the body. This letting go is part of the dying process; the physical body, etheric body, soul and I slowly separate from each other. This means that perception becomes more body-free; we see this, for instance, in near-death experiences, during which those dying may see themselves floating above their body.

The senses become more sensitive, and it is of great importance to take this into account. If we allow those dying to have too many sense impressions they may experience it as pain, and it may distract them from the actual process. And yet it is the senses which, with the 'right' observation, may be helpful to come back into the body for a moment, in order to be able to make the last essential observations before leaving the earth behind. The ways in which this last phase of life can be made valuable to the dying person differ for each individual.

In the morning hours the wondrous phenomenon occurred that all sensory impressions were extremely fine and sharp for Paul. It was as if the soul adopted a body of an infinitely more tender and refined structure. In taste and smell all kinds of memory pictures arose in him with great subtlety; he became so sensitive to light that he had to wear dark glasses, although he still observed everything that happened around him quite precisely. He reacted to each gesture, to the lightest touch, to each whispered word – yes, his hearing was so sharp that he understood word for word a whispered conversation I had with the physician in the farthest corner of the room.

I was familiar with this phenomenon in dying people, but I had never witnessed it to such a great extent. And yet, by that time Paul's body had become useless and could no longer serve him. He had not eaten for days, his kidneys didn't work at all anymore, his breathing was very shallow, his pulse hardly perceptible – and still the spirit found a way to manifest itself with total clarity in this irretrievable and helpless wreckage, with the finest perceptive capacities, the most noble sense of clear self-observation.

– *Eeden,* Pauls ontwaken, *p. 58*

Hearing

Noises sound much louder for dying people than for others. Things like running faucets, squeaking or banging doors, loud footsteps, shrill voices, and the like may be almost unbearable. It is therefore good to make sure that the surroundings of a dying person have an atmosphere of peace and quiet. Be conscious of what you are doing. Don't thoughtlessly turn on a radio or TV. Ask yourself if you yourself are perhaps afraid of silence.

Hearing remains intact the longest of all the senses. When someone is on the point of dying, or is in a coma, we have the tendency to talk about the patient in their presence because we think that they cannot hear us anyway. But very likely this person is experiencing more and more of what we think and feel, because the spiritual world is already penetrating into earthly life. It is important to be aware of this because otherwise we might hinder the dying person in their process of disengaging.

Vision

What does the room of the dying person look like? I often hear healthy people say that a patient's room should not be sombre, but nice and inviting. But is that for the bystanders or for the patient? What does the patient prefer? A dying person experiences colour around them more intensely than others. Take this into account.

Some dying people find blank walls a soothing relief. Others dislike that and want something on the wall, for instance, a real painting or reproduction that conveys a true, living image. The human being on the threshold looks for meaning. A physician had the following experience:

An 89-year-old man decided to deal with his pneumonia with an anthroposophic therapy, and not with antibiotics. One day he was doing so badly that he received the last rites. During the ritual he had an extraordinary inner experience, and was subsequently healed. During a check-up three months later it turned out that lung cancer had been the cause of the pneumonia.

Three years later he felt that he had come to the end of his life. He called his doctor and told him that he was going to stay in bed and would only drink. The doctor supported this decision. Later he realised that because the patient was also deaf, his communication with the world around him through the senses had become extremely limited – no taste, no smell, hardly any hearing. He decided to bring him a large reproduction of Rembrandt's *Man in Armour* – the man with the helmet, red mantle and spear – in order that at least there would be a beautiful impression for the eye.

Two days later the patient got up and started eating again. The observation of the painting by Rembrandt had brought him back into incarnation so that continued life was possible again. During the next few days he had some profound meetings with people. Two weeks later the doctor was called again for a final leave-taking. Three hours later the patient died.

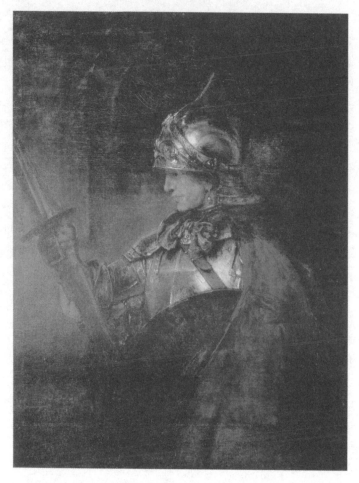

Rembrandt van Rijn, Man in Armour, *1655, Kelvingrove Art Gallery and Museum, Glasgow.*

Smell

We may be overwhelmed by smells, but we cannot say: 'I don't want to smell anything.' We have to breathe in, which compels us to take in something from outside. The primal aspect of smelling is its compelling characteristic. When we are overwhelmed by a scent, we tend to lose ourselves. A sign of this is that after a while we don't smell anything anymore – the scent is in us. Someone else has to come into the room and say: 'This place stinks' or 'It smells so good here.'

For this reason keep food smells away from a dying person. They may even smell what the neighbours are cooking. Don't use perfume, aftershave, scented soap, in brief, anything that has a scent. This may even include flowers.

> He wanted nothing pretty or colourful around him. The only things he could tolerate were white flowers without scent. 'They are so beautiful!' he would whisper. And when lilac and yellow flowers were added to them he said: 'I would have liked to have them taken out, but I didn't dare to ask.' He was afraid to offend those who had put them there for him.
>
> White flowers without scent was what he wanted. This meant that he could no longer bear worldly colours and scents. He wanted to prepare himself for a higher, more delicate receptivity.
> – *Eeden,* Pauls ontwaken, *pp. 42f*

Taste

When we eat, we take care of the life processes in the body so that a healthy unity is preserved. But in the dying process the reverse occurs: the life processes want to detach themselves. For this reason a dying person often has no appetite. Nourishment is no longer needed, for eating tends to connect us with the earth again. The saying 'eating makes you strong' no longer holds true.

However, good, regular meals are important for people who mourn and give help, because by their sympathy for the dying person they tend to loosen their connection with the earth, and because they also 'die a little,' they can lose their appetite.

If we try to help a dying person with tasty food, it is often hard to accept that they may hardly touch the meal. But don't reproach them. Through the attention with which you prepare the food you add creative forces. Even though the dying person may not eat it, or just take a small bite, they still receive your love. Besides the attention with which it is prepared it is also important to consider the quality of the food. A thoughtfully arranged diet of organic or biodynamic food may influence the quality of life and the lucidity of spirit during the illness.

Try to stimulate the warmth processes in the body of the dying person. Avoid cooled food or drink, or food prepared in a microwave. Although the food may be heated up that way, the manner of heating is in fact cold; no real heat is involved.

If the dying person still has a last wish relating to eating, such as tasting something they used to enjoy so much one last time, by all means, gratify that wish. It is often a wish from memory, not out of appetite. Even if they take just one little bite, the satisfaction of a momentary connection with the earthly is also nourishment. Set the patient at ease if they do not eat everything – that was not the point, was it?

Drinking will have to be carefully arranged in coordination with the wishes of the patient and their need for fluids. If the patient does not want to take in anything anymore, the professional judgment of a physician and loving care for the individuality of the dying person are needed to respond to this in the right way. Thirst may often no longer play a role, and a little moisture on the lips by a wet cloth with a little ice in it will often suffice. Lip balm may prevent excessively dry lips and lemon sticks may mitigate dryness in the mouth.

The sense of warmth

Warmth is the experience that is closest to us. Feeling for warmth and cold is most emphatically present. Even when people with dementia can hardly name anything anymore they can still accurately tell whether they are cold or warm. During the dying phase cold often occurs, mostly in the body and especially at its extremities: in feet, legs, hands and tip of the nose. Physical unrest in dying people is caused by cold legs; this hinders the process of letting go, just as cold feet prevent many people from falling asleep. Warming them up again brings quiet and makes the dying process less stressful. See also Chapter 13 on external therapy.

Coldness in the soul may also impede the dying process, and for bystanders it may indicate that there is still something that has to happen. In that case you need to search for something that 'warms' the person in their connection with the end of their life.

The sense of touch

Touch is separation and connection at the same time.
– *Novalis*

A baby becomes conscious of itself through caresses, warmth and love. To a dying person physical touch may also be important. It conveys the experience of the security of the body, even when the body no longer feels comfortable. Touch gives us a twofold experience: we not only feel the boundaries of what we touch, but also our own boundaries. To touch and to be touched generates an inner movement, but there must be no hint of haste, possessiveness or selfishness, for then it is unbearable. Touching creates an intimate connection in greatest freedom: two souls carry each other. On an inner soul level we can create a space to explore the I of the other and to be touched by the personality of the other.

If touch leaves the other unfree, for example, because you really don't want them to leave you, holding the hand may be experienced as compulsion, and may impede the process of letting go. A dying person is frequently so sensitive that thoughtless caresses can cause anguish.

Visions on the deathbed

There was a physics professor who had worked with quantum mechanics all his life, and did not believe in a spiritual world, let alone a life after death. His last words on his deathbed, while he looked up in amazement, were, 'Yes, the spiritual world exists!' Then he died.

A germ of a new consciousness of eternity, a budding awareness of a level in ourselves that transcends transient, material existence, may sprout on the deathbed. Identification with outer life disappears, and consciousness makes a connection with our higher self – a radical change of consciousness. The connection with our own essential core is experienced more intensely. Identification with our outer, physical state of consciousness splits off and becomes, in a certain sense, unreal. The sensory delusion in which we often live dissolves and shows us its reality and its meaning or meaninglessness.

We become conscious of the fact that the eternal and transitory worlds are woven together. Close to death the veil is sometimes briefly lifted, and it is given to us to have a quick look into the spiritual world. It is like an announcement of an awakening in deeper layers of our being.

Prior to dying we are often shown how we receive assistance from departed souls dear to us with whom we had a connection during our lives.

> My great-grandmother was a very religious woman, but about life after death she was at a total loss and simply couldn't believe it. Just before her passing she said suddenly: 'John, is it you? Is it then true after all?' Then she died. John was her son who had died a few years earlier.
> – *Roos*

It is important that physicians and others who are present when someone dies are aware of the significance of these visions for the dying person and for those they leave behind. In the first place the way in which the dying person crosses the threshold is important for themselves; for the surviving relatives it can be a consolation, and maybe it can give them a sense of the existence of life after death. Whether a dying person has such visions may depend on the medications they are receiving.

Karlis Osis and Erlendur Haraldsson, two psychologists who have collected many cases of visions in the hour of death, have done research in this area. They have described that such deathbed visions are very similar to near-death experiences. A dying patient who has suffered pain for several days and then suddenly feels no pain or discomfort is a phenomenon that can also be observed with people who have had a near-death experience. In deathbed visions, as in near-death experiences, there are also frequent images of other worlds and of conversations with people who have passed away earlier.

Osis and Haraldsson observed that the deathbed visions they collected came mostly from patients to whom no sedatives had been administered and who, a few hours before death, were still lucid. The contents of the visions showed great differences, but many visions spoke of relatives and friends who had died earlier and who, according to the dying person, had come to take them with them.

Here follows a vision related by a nurse who was sitting at the deathbed of a forty-year-old man:

> He had had no sedatives and was fully conscious of everything.
> He did have a low temperature. He was religious and believed
> in a life after death. We were expecting that he would die soon,
> and this did indeed happen. He asked us to pray for him. In
> his room was a stairway that led to a second floor. Suddenly
> he called out: 'Look, the angels are descending. The glass has
> fallen and is broken.' We were shocked and looked at the stairs
> where a glass of water was standing on one of the steps. While
> we were looking, the glass, without any demonstrable cause,
> was shattered into a thousand pieces. It didn't fall, it simply
> exploded. Of course, we could not see the angels. The patient's
> face showed a peaceful and happy expression, and in the next
> moment he breathed his last. Even after his death his face
> retained the peaceful expression.
> – *Morse,* Closer to the Light

Occasionally it may also happen to the next of kin that a corner of the veil is lifted. Knowing that we are being expected when we die can be a great source of strength and courage.

When my father was dying, about two weeks before his passing,
my mother sat a little away from him and looked at him while
he was sleeping. As twilight was falling outside and she could
no longer precisely distinguish his features, behind the head of
the bed a golden light source grew that shone over his whole
body. In that soft light my mother saw a circle of kneeling
figures, dressed like monks with pointed hoods, who were
doing something with him. My mother had the impression
that they were busy loosening my father from his earthly body.
After some time one of these figures looked up, and she saw
the familiar face of a friend who has passed away shortly before.
The next moment the image dissolved.
– *Joyce*

It may also happen that on the threshold of death a person receives
strength from someone who died earlier, in order to remain on the
earth. Sometimes even those around the person become aware of this.
Mariska relates the following:

There I am. I am standing at the deathbed of my husband Luke,
who was then 34. Half an hour earlier, when life seemed to be
taking its usual course, I had a call from the police, had to pick up
the children from school and leave them with friends, and drive
to the hospital to hear that my husband had probably had a stroke,
was in a deep coma and would most likely die. I immediately called
relatives and friends who would take care of the kids. My parents,
parents-in-law and one of Luke's brothers came immediately.

Yes, there I stand together with my brother-in-law and we
both look at Luke and see the deathly pallor of his face showing
that he is more dead than alive. Motionless we look at him. It
is so incredibly intense that even tears hold back. I look at my
husband, the love of my life; my brother-in-law looks at his
brother and playmate.

Suddenly something changes in the atmosphere; I am surprised, for it feels like light and hope. Gradually, I see a kind of veil-like apparition, and I very distinctly feel the presence of Ina, Luke's sister who had passed away about a year before. I literally hear her speak, 'You don't belong here yet, you have no business here. You have things to do and to finish there. Go away!' Typical for the way Ina used to be!

I let the whole thing come over me like a kind of cloak, and remember that in some way it made me happy. Quietly we leave the room again to let Luke's parents be with him and say goodbye to him. After about ten minutes a physician rushes up to us and tells us that there is a change in Luke's condition and that there is some hope. But he wants to send him to a specialist hospital. We race to the other place, Luke has surgery, he lies in a coma for a time, but the risk of death is becoming less and less.

During one of the many nights of waiting and watching, I am standing on the balcony with my brother-in-law and ask him with some hesitation whether he also sensed Ina's presence in that special moment. He answers with a whole-hearted yes. We have never talked about it since then, but we are both certain that she was there.

After a very long illness Luke remains seriously handicapped. He lives in an institution and I support him whenever I can and often try to be with him. Very often when I am with him I sense Ina's presence; I know she is there, he is not alone. He is being carried by her from the spiritual world and by us here on earth.

In conclusion, I want to relate that my sister-in-law, Ina, died of cancer at age 39, and left a family behind with four children and a husband. A terrible situation in the process of which she proved to be the strongest. My husband, Luke, gave her tremendous support during her illness. They had long and remarkable conversations, and he shared much of her suffering. In her search for the right way through this illness Luke was there for her, and in their talks they were able to develop insights.

In the end, Ina had to let go of life, and she knew it. Luke, however, was not yet able to accept that, and could no longer really listen to her. He had but one great goal, which was that she would remain alive; that she would be able to complete her path here and that she would not have to leave her husband and, especially, her children. It was a shock for Luke when he suddenly realised that she was going to die, that he really had to take leave of his sister, and that he did not have to fight for her life here anymore.

When Ina died the whole family stood arm in arm around her, and her husband and children were lying in her arms. The connection was beautiful. The year that followed was one of mourning for everyone. For Luke it meant that he had to find a form for his taking leave of his sister, and that he could let go of his battle and guilt feelings. This was a difficult, but also salutary process. Eventually he made an altar with a pretty picture and fresh flowers and often stood before it, praying. Luke so wanted to feel her and have contact with her, but for the first time in his life he really found himself. Just over a year later Luke had his stroke.

Despite everything, the daily troubles and all the suffering I have to bear every day, I feel I am a blessed person. Through all the little and great miracles I feel confidence in life itself, and through these genuine and unique experiences I feel connected with the spiritual world, and I feel carried. The following verse gives me strength every day:

The wishes of the soul are springing,
The deeds of the will are thriving,
The fruits of life are maturing.

I feel my fate,
My fate finds me,
I feel my star,
My star finds me,
I feel my goals in life,
My goals in life are finding me.
My soul and the great world are one.
Life grows more radiant about me,
Life grows more arduous for me,
Grows more abundant within me.
– *Steiner,* Verses and Meditations, *p. 113*

The intuition of animals

The human being knows and the animal knows,
But the human being is the only one
Who knows that he knows.
– *Teilhard de Chardin*

The intuition of animals is mind-boggling, especially in cases of death and mourning, or when their owner or family members are in danger. For that reason they must certainly not be forgotten in this book.

Jean Parker who lives in Peterborough, noticed that something unusual was going on when she arrived home from work one afternoon and was surprised to find her cat Timmy waiting for her; he habitually slept on her son's bed all day. 'He kept meowing very pitifully and I thought he was in physical pain, but no amount of fussing him would calm him down at all. To cut a long story short, at 8.15 pm I learned my son had had a very bad road accident and was in intensive care at Addenbrooke's Hospital in Cambridge and was in danger

of losing his life. My son was in that unit for seven weeks in a coma. Timmy would not go into his bedroom. But then one evening Timmy ran straight into my son's room, jumped on the bed and began purring with deep pleasure. That was the day my son came out of his coma and began to get back to life again.'
– *Sheldrake,* The Sense of Being Stared At, *pp. 78f*

A young single farmer one day fell down dead on his farm. His dog, a cross between a shepherd dog and a Rottweiler, was always with him. Wherever he went, the dog was there too. The man was taken in an ambulance to a hospital, where he was pronounced dead. His body was to lie in state in the farmhouse. When the undertaker came with the body to the farm gate, the dog was locked up according to the family. They had asked that the body be taken through the property, past the stables and the machines. The family walked behind the hearse, the undertaker in front of it. Imagine people's surprise when they saw that the dog had broken out of its pen and was walking quietly beside the undertaker, at the same pace, across the whole property. It didn't bark or growl. Upon arrival at the front door the dog lay down and quietly watched how the farmer's body was carried into the house.
– *Liesbeth*

A friend told me of her mother's cat that was present when she received the last rites.

My mother was going to receive the last rites. She was very weak and it was thought that she had not much longer to live after the major surgery she had undergone. In the house where she lived with seven other people, a few family members, the inhabitants and a few good friends came together to attend the ritual.

Just before the priest wanted to begin, the cat slipped into the room and sat beside me. The cat actually never used to sit with me, but now it pressed its body against me and, quivering lightly, was there throughout the ceremony. Afterward it disappeared again. It must have sensed that something important was happening to its mistress, and wanted to be there.

The cat was a good indicator of the condition of my mother. When she was not doing well, it looked kind of dull; when mother got better again, the cat's coat looked nice and glossy. They had a very special connection, those two.

And finally two experiences of the connection between human beings and animals, and the fidelity an animal can have even across the threshold of death.

From one day to the next Nino, your cat, refused to eat. I got a lot of delicacies for him, but he refused to eat them. I even put them in his mouth, but he spat them out. The vet fed him intravenously – in vain, for at home he continued to reject all food. Then, exactly a month after you, he died. He refused to remain behind without you.
– *Tony, speaking to his wife who had died*

Pivo is my neighbours' dog across the street. Pivo had had a few accidents and my husband, John, had helped taking care of him. Pivo loved John.

On February 13, 2004 my husband died. Four to five weeks after his death I clearly heard footsteps in the hallway upstairs while I was lying in bed at night. This was repeated every night. John was always the last to go to bed, he would lock the front door and turn off the lights. The sound of the footsteps made me restless and I wondered if I was imagining it.

Pivo had stayed with us sometimes, and now I asked the neighbours if he could stay with me again for a few days. He was lying on my bed as usual when I heard the footsteps again. Pivo sat up straight, growled and went downstairs. Since then, whenever he was with me at night, he only wanted to sleep downstairs.

A few months later I took Pivo with me on a visit to the urn with John's ashes. When we came to the entrance of the cemetery he started pulling on the leash. I took him off the leash and he flew away like an arrow. I followed. He went straight to the place where the urn was standing, put his paws on the wall, started to bark loudly and kept sniffing and licking the stone. I felt the tears streaming down my face. I wanted to leave, but couldn't get Pivo to come with me. He finally barked loudly again and then suddenly walked away.

When I take him to the cemetery now, he runs to the stone and licks it as if he wants to show he is there again.

After we had been to the cemetery Pivo spent the night with me again. Once more I heard the footsteps; Pivo also heard them, but he never left my bed. I think John wanted to let us know that he had seen us. I hope that when Pivo dies my husband will be waiting for him, because Pivo will then be with his great friend.

– *Jannie*

10

THE LANGUAGE OF IMAGES AT THE THRESHOLD

Bert Voorhoeve

'I am going to move soon,' said an old farmer
who was walking on his land with his daughter.
The daughter thought the father was talking
nonsense, for there had never been any question
of moving. A few days later the father died;
he had spoken of his approaching death.

People who go through a crisis in their life, people who are seriously ill or dying, and people with a near-death experience often use images to express their experiences. Such images reflect a reality that cannot be described in the words of our everyday language. It is important for people who care for ill and dying persons to be receptive to this imagery, so that they are able to understand it, and also speak it. Help for those dying asks for closeness to the other and for following them in their images, as well as creating images for them that can give consolation and courage.

Symbols, parables, poetry, fairytales and Bible stories may help go through the largely invisible processes around dying. Empathy, intuition and imagination are needed to find those images that can give inner strength, and with which they can identify while having certain experiences. It is therefore most important to listen closely to the images a dying person experiences and relates to. These may help us, since we may assume that they are expressions of inner experiences on the threshold between life and death.

In this regard it is helpful if during our life we develop a feeling for imagery as it lives, for instance, in poetry, fairytales, the Bible, nature, and in our own life.

Crises open the heart for images

If in the course of life we develop a sense for the language of imagery, we can find that especially in crisis situations caused by problems, illness, loss, leave-taking or dying, images may have a consoling and encouraging effect. That is because images can throw a surprisingly new light on difficult life situations. Especially if we are thrown back onto ourselves we may become very receptive to them.

Some time ago I was in a deep valley, both literally and figuratively, because I was having lung problems and was staying for a few months in an asthma clinic in Davos, Switzerland. Looking out from my room I saw the snowy rock face of the mountains that were often hidden in clouds. Sometimes you couldn't see anything through a thick fog or snowfall that would last for days on end. It could be depressing.

One Sunday morning I opened the curtains and was deeply touched by an incredible spectacle. On the top of the mountain I saw the golden glow of the sun that was just rising behind it. The wind at the top blew clouds of snow about. The sparkling crystals of snow that were dancing in the light of the first sunrays. The snow-covered pine trees on the mountain also looked as if they were made of crystal because the sun was shining through the snowy branches.

This experience grew into an image: when you are caught in a valley you should 'open the curtains,' look outside and let yourself be surprised by what you see there. I experienced it as a gift; I felt myself coming to life again after a period of depression that had given me a feeling of wading through a swamp, hidden in thick fog.

This sunrise also awoke me again to the power of images, and I resolved to tell my fellow patients a fairytale. I had been impressed by the stories my fellow patients had told about their way through the valley – their struggles with illness and the side effects of their medications. When one of the patients was celebrating a birthday I overcame my reserve and told Grimm's fairytale of the devil with the three golden hairs. In the space, which was dominated by an enormous television screen, you could hear a pin drop. After I told the fairytale I was moved by the gratitude that came to me. For days people mentioned the fairytale and told me what an impression it had made on them. Someone said, 'Such a fairytale is really much nicer than those TV films we are always watching. With that kind of story you can form your own images.'

Images around dying

Every day my mother made the rounds through the nursing home with her walker. But then she fell and broke a hip. She received morphine for the pain, and when my wife and I came to visit her she was lying in her room, unresponsive. No contact of any kind was possible. It was clear that my mother would not be alive much longer. My wife and I stayed with her. We told her Grimm's fairytale of the girl who gives away all she has, and then receives a new shift and stars from heaven. We told my mother that she could now let go of everything just like the girl in the fairytale. Halfway through the story I couldn't continue anymore; I became too emotional. My wife continued the fairytale and then we saw, deeply moved, three tears coming out of my mother's eyes. We had the feeling that we had contact through the images of the fairytale. A few hours later my mother died.

The story gives a picture of separation, as the girl successively gives away all her food and clothing to others, with the result that a receptivity could grow for the spiritual world, which we enter when we die. The fairytale tells us that we can replace our earthly clothes by heavenly clothes. When we have nothing left, and stand there naked, we are able to receive the heavenly robe of the 'finest linen,' and the stars of heaven become part of our new existence. Thus outer poverty changes into inner riches.

A few months before her death a girl of thirteen wrote the poem *Moving*. The ending was as follows:

> The TV, the plants and so on,
> Everything has now been packed;
> For the last time the fire is put out
> (I had chopped the wood for it).
> Then... silence;
> A tear wells up; I say:
> Goodbye best house that ever was,
> Goodbye, perhaps, perhaps.
> – *from Stolp,* Als dood te vroeg komt

After the death of her young daughter a mother said: 'Fortunately she never knew it.' She was unable to talk about death with her daughter. The latter asked shortly before she died: 'Mom, could you please read me a fairytale?' She wanted Andersen's fairytale of *The Little Match Girl*. It is about a girl who is dying in cold surroundings, but it also speaks of light and warmth when she experiences that on the border between life and death she is born into a new existence. The question of the girl was not understood by those around her.

Images are also important because they can express fearful or threatening experiences. In his book, Hans Stolp describes that a girl had dreamed of a dragon. She dreamt that she was floating away from land in a little boat. Her father, mother, little brother and sister were standing on land. Suddenly a dragon came out of the water and wanted to grasp her. Stolp describes how he tried to help the girl by following her pictures. He asked, 'Where is the dragon? Do you dare touch him? Or pet him? Do you dare sit on him?' Through this game of fantasy the girl quieted down and overcame her fear.

The importance of fairytales

In my room I have a small red box containing a ball of golden thread. This ball has gone through many hands. I let the ball go around the circle when I tell a fairytale to a group. Everyone can then relate how they experienced the golden thread in the fairytale. And the golden thread that then connected people with each other is a picture of the golden thread of the life of each person, which was briefly experienced as common to all.

The ball of golden thread gives a picture of the power of fairytales. It is the ball that an old man or woman gives to the boy or girl, the prince or princess who went out into the world and lost their way. When you throw the ball ahead of you, it shows you the way. It is also Ariadne's thread that showed Theseus the way back out of the labyrinth where he had to defeat a monster.

When you tell or read a fairytale you hand the listener this golden thread of life. The thread may become tangled or get into a knot, or it may break. Fairytales tell us that we can find a new golden thread if we have lost our way. Fairytales speak in pictures about human life. They can console us because we can recognise in them our own grief, hope, doubt, fear, courage, anger, despair, optimism.

In fairytales we can experience that despite all the troubles in life there is hope, even if we are down and out, if we have lost our way in a dark forest, if we are skirting an abyss or are caught in a swamp, and if we have to take leave of someone who is dear to us. In the dark wood there is a little light, by the abyss or the swamp lives someone who can help, who consoles us and has a fire where we can warm ourselves. Also if we have to say goodbye and are grieving, there are people who can console us and give us the feeling that we are not alone.

In fairytales 'the child' and 'the wise one' come together. When we tell or read a fairytale to an ill or dying person we speak to 'the child' and 'the wise one' in them, the forces of openness, open-mindedness, wonder, faith and trust that grow from deep wisdom obtained through life experience. That is the great power of fairytales.

What we still had by nature as a child, living with images, we lost as we grew into adulthood. We can try to find the child in ourselves again.

11

MUSIC FOR TERMINALLY ILL PEOPLE

Hilly Bol

Music goes beyond words. What cannot be expressed in words takes refuge in music. This is why I find writing about music so difficult. How can I find words for what music is? And how can I convey something about the role music may play in the last phase of life? Of course, we may write about melody, beat and rhythm, about tempo and harmony – the various musical elements. That doesn't need to be bare and analytical; it also offers potential for images and analogies. But the essence and inner power of music dwell in the music itself. Perhaps we can trace some of that in the stories that follow.

Music: mirror of earthly life

There are so many kinds of music, so many forms, so many colours – all these different kinds together seem to form a metaphor for everything that meets us in our earthly life. Our mutual relationships, our feelings and emotions, our ideas, they can all be found in music. Our experiences in nature around us, the woods, the flowers, the ocean, a waterfall, fire, clouds – they can be reflected in music. There is music to dance to; there is music to sing by; there is music to be very quiet.

Music may touch us deeply. Music may comfort us. Music can upset us and can also calm us down. The Bible tells us that David played his harp when Saul fell into a depression. In the early Middle Ages the monks in the monastery of Cluny sang for one who was on his deathbed, sometimes for many hours. And all over the world mothers sing lullabies to their child.

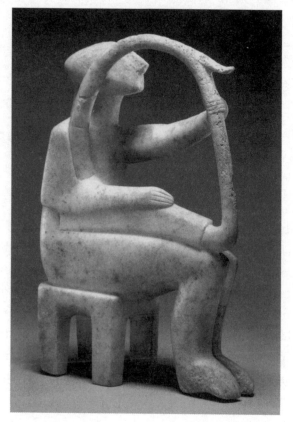

Harp player of the Cyclades, *c. 2500 BC, Getty Villa, Malibu, California.*

Music during the last part of life

Not so very long ago people who were dying in hospitals were put in a room somewhere out of the way. Fortunately, in more recent years much has changed in the way terminal and dying patients are cared for. This is particularly obvious in hospice and home care, as well as in some nursing homes. There is much more respect for people's own identity and the great differences in their wishes for their last moments on earth.

Music is slowly finding a place in palliative care, albeit still a modest one. Music can be chosen with love and care to be played on a CD player. Some kinds of music are not appropriate, maybe too busy, too much, too complex, but even that is not true for everyone. Then there is live music. I know of daughters who sang at the deathbed of their mother; of a son who played his cello; of a woman who was in the Salvation Army and wanted so much to hear a trumpet again.

On a small scale it has also become possible to offer music live. On a small scale, for music therapy still has a long way to develop. When music is played live, it is possible to adapt how it is played to the moment and the situation. It is often quite possible to use the breathing rhythm of the ill or dying person as a guide in the decision as to what to play and how. Everything we can observe through our senses can help us in choosing the music. There may also be room for the music of silence. Then a word may be spoken that still needed to be spoken, a gesture may be made that still needed to be made; and the silence may deepen further and further. Thus music touches body, soul and spirit, not only of the one who is dying, but also of the others who are present, family members, friends, and caregivers.

The nurse came out of one of the rooms in the hospice and said to me: 'I don't know what it is, but she is not doing well. It is as if she is stuck somehow. Maybe music can help her.' I was just walking in the hallway after I had played for one of the other people. The nurse went back into the room to consult with the husband, who was in complete agreement to give it a try. They also asked Mrs Z. herself, but she was not able to react.

Uncertainly I went in, not knowing how it would be and how she would react, because I had not played for her before. Mrs Z. was lying in her bed in semi-darkness, and her husband sat on a chair close by. The atmosphere felt oppressive. Mrs Z. was lying on her back, breathing fast and superficially. Her eyes were open but when I came closer to make contact, her gaze was empty. She couldn't speak. I briefly held her hand which felt cold and a little damp. Her pulse was very fast but still had some strength.

'I have come to play some music on my harp for you; maybe that will help a little.' Mr Z. moved uncomfortably in his chair.

I didn't know what was going on, but perhaps I did not need to know. The word stagnation arose in me. Seated at the harp I followed her breathing and silently asked what was needed. Movement?

Tentatively: one sound, then cautiously another, the second, right next to the first one. Then back to the first, a little louder. Slowly the sounds followed each other in the space until there was a distinguishable stream that began to fill the room. The melody became recognisable, a $\frac{3}{4}$ rhythm, an old Celtic song, to my surprise with quite a strict rhythm. I rarely play this music so rhythmically as I did then. I kept playing like this for about ten minutes, with little variations, and sang softly along with an oo-sound. The oo-sound is cautious, but also reassuring.

Mrs Z. moved a leg; a moment later we heard a sigh. Her breathing became a little deeper and slower. Again she moved her leg. Then came a little moan. Mr Z. took her hand. He was sitting still on his chair. The music gradually became quieter and moved from minor to major. Was it to create more space? We left that strict rhythm and moved into more flowing forms. Space for all there may be, here in this room, with this dying woman and her husband. Melodious sounds with always the same descending pattern of notes, repeated time after time, like a temporary little anchor in uncertain waters. Again I sang along, now with an a-sound, broader.

Slowly and quietly I rounded it off. There was more space now in Mrs Z.'s breath. When I took leave we momentarily looked into each other's eyes. It felt different then, less oppressive. A few hours later she quietly passed away.

Sensing your way to music

Just as at birth and at giving birth, a mystery unfolds at death. It always fills me with great respect for the secrets of life and death. What a privilege to be able to witness this, like a kind of midwife.

In terminal care and during the process of dying, music can work as a supporting and soothing remedy, both for the dying person and for the family members. Music and silence create something like a riverbed, which every time takes a different course.

When I look back on Mrs Z., who had become stuck in her difficult struggle, it seems possible that it was caused by a paralysing fear. Do I know this? I am never sure, but that her dying process was stagnating was something the nurses and I later agreed on. Mrs Z.'s last hours were calmer. Maybe she would have come to this change without music, but we all had the impression that it had helped her.

Music can work on us in many different ways. Rhythmical music stimulates us to movement. Sometimes you can't control your legs anymore and feel that you want to dance. With the dying I don't often use such outspoken rhythms; if I do, I do it very carefully, for it can quickly become too much. I almost never use a $\frac{2}{4}$ or $\frac{4}{4}$ beat. The $\frac{3}{4}$ rhythm gives a more flowing movement; just think of a waltz. To learn what influence a particular rhythm has on us, we can move with it so that we feel what it does to the body.

Music is born from silence. In that silence I often ask: 'What is needed?' Is the situation asking for musical confirmation of what is there – music as resonance of what is occurring in the moment? Or can music be used as a 'counterforce' as in the case of Mrs Z.? The choice is not always easy, but while playing it is important to continue listening and, as it were, keep feeling your way. For Mrs Z. the music was a clear invitation to come into movement; she visibly came back into her body, just once more, the last time, for a deep farewell to that familiar, but also arduous, painful, sick body.

So much can happen in those last weeks of life, such intensive processes may have to be gone through. I have come to realise this more and more and it has left a deep impression on me, in my personal life and also by playing the harp for terminally ill and dying people.

She was a 74-year-old widow, had had lung cancer for some time, and the hospital could do no more for her. Unfortunately, hospitals are not always good at giving palliative care; it is as if hospital care and the care for a dying person take place in different octaves. Due to metastasis Mrs B. broke a hip and had surgery for it, and subsequently could no longer manage life at home. She received hospice care and her sons and daughter-in-law frequently visited her.

I had already played a few times for her. She clearly indicated that she liked it. Slowly but surely she got worse. I agreed with her daughter-in-law that I would play for her one evening when both daughters-in-law and a grandchild would be there. We formed a circle around the bed. Consciously or unconsciously, we participated in a ritual. Mrs B. was lying half on her side; she had become so small. Speech was no longer possible. Her daughter-in-law moistened her lips and gave her a little bit of water. The music was simple, a lullaby that felt like a combination of softness and strength. Suddenly she said with a loud voice, 'Wonderful!' And we thought that she could not speak anymore.

Three days later I played for her for the last time. She was even smaller and skinnier and looked like a feather. Her breathing was audible for some time, then almost gone. For a moment she was alone. Listening, looking, feeling, I asked in silence what was there – it was like the changing tides – sometimes she was there, then again she was not. Was she practising her transition?

When later I was asking myself why I played the way I did – much alternation between rhythm and free form – I realised that it was because of those movements between here and there, between in and out of her body. The music reflected that.

That same night she died very peacefully.

Such a ritual can deepen the process of leave-taking. It did so for the wife of a dying man. She had difficulties expressing herself. When the last sounds died away she said with profound emotion and from the bottom of her heart: 'You may go.' For many years she had taken care of her husband with great dedication, as Parkinson's disease was making him more and more into an invalid. Then the time came when she couldn't handle it anymore. A few weeks later she had to entrust the care to others. It was a big step. And now again, a big step to say this out of the very ground of her being.

Or that time when the husband was sitting far from the bed of his wife. With the children and their partners we were sitting in a circle. I didn't dare ask him to come closer; I didn't know why he was sitting there so by himself. He didn't seem approachable. The music was at the request of his wife, but every time the music stopped he moved his chair a little. The children walked to their mother or held each other in consoling gestures. Again the husband moved a little. After half an hour he sat beside his wife's bed and briefly held her hand. Words were not needed. The music did it.

I will never forget Anna. She was just thirty, but had contracted breast cancer as a very young woman. She had had all kinds of treatments. Two weeks ago, she was in intensive care because of metastasis into the brain. Then things got a little better. She was placed in hospice care and was expected to die soon.

Her brother and his wife were visiting, and it was quiet in the room. I played for her a piece of old Gregorian music. Then there was silence and she said she wanted to sit up. She began to speak. When she was lying in intensive care and was in a serious condition, she had an experience she wanted to share with her brother and sister-in-law. She spoke of the wonderful light and of perfect love. In this near-death experience she had been close to the end. Through the music all of this came to the surface again. She had not told anyone before. We were all touched by her story.

A week later I was in the same care facility and heard from a nurse that Anna was doing remarkably well. When I entered her room, she was sitting on a chair beside her bed. She smiled and began to explain to me that she did not want to listen to harp music anymore. 'It brings me very close to death, and I believe that I am allowed to live a while longer.' It was nice to talk to her again.

Anna lived for a long time after that.

Anna herself was able to indicate that she had no need for this music. But what about people who can no longer communicate their wishes? One experience that taught me a lot was the time when I came into Liz's room; I had played for her a number of times. She was lying there with her eyes closed; she had lost a lot of weight and seemed almost transparent. It was completely silent in her room and around her. This silence was sacred. I sensed that I could and need no longer play for her.

Every time it is a question of feeling my way – when and how can music be a support, and create a channel for all that is there? When is restraint demanded? When is energy the right thing?

I am grateful for the many possibilities to consult with others, in the first place with the people in the care facilities, but also with the relatives and with all those who work there and sometimes say to me, 'Would you play something for us?' In this way music becomes embedded in the care for the dying. I am also grateful for the harp and singing training I received at the School for Music Thanatology of Therese Schroeder-Sheker (Chalice of Repose Project, Missoula, Montana). Without the foundation that was laid there I would not have been able to begin this work.

I do not want to shortchange those who play for sick or dying people with other instruments. The lyre and also other instruments are used to play for dying people. Hopefully more exchange of experiences and new initiatives will make it possible to gradually expand the potential for music for the ill and the dying.

12

ARTISTIC THERAPY

Marieke Udo de Haes-Mulder

In a terminal period, we may distinguish a palliative phase and terminal phase. The palliative phase runs from three months to six weeks before death. The subsequent phase is usually called terminal, although it may still be divided into a pre-terminal and a terminal phase. In this last phase the patient is usually bedridden and cannot paint.

I have had the privilege to paint with a dear friend in Bulgaria during the last months of his life. When I was there he had just been told that he had an incurable illness, cancer of the liver. This message was for him reason to deny his illness with great force. He, and everyone around him, acted as though it did not exist. For me it was difficult to participate in this phase of denial, especially because I had limited time. I had a strong feeling that guided artistic exercises could have great significance for him in this condition of shock.

When I cautiously offered to work together with him he reacted with enthusiasm. For a number of weeks we painted intensively every day, we worked with pastel, and spoke of the unexpected turn in his life. I had to make a choice between directing the artistic exercises more toward the illness, the liver disorder, or to the mourning process. If the latter, I would have to give more confrontational exercises.

First I decided to ask him to paint a so-called free exercise, an exercise with all colours on which no influence from outside of any kind is made. In this exercise the breakdown of his body came to expression. Because of the evident picture of the stage of his illness I then gave him guided exercises that related to the process of the illness.

Of course, due to the various colour moods and experiences intensive conversations also began to take place. He was extremely happy to finally have someone with whom he could speak about his condition and, eventually, also about his death. For in Bulgaria, family and friends do not speak about dying, loss, mourning; they show no grief – all of that is just not done – everything is kept from the sick person as much as possible. After all, it is important that there be joy around the person for as long as they are still there. A good idea perhaps, but difficult to realise!

A month after I had returned home, my Bulgarian friend peacefully died.

When I look back on this precious encounter, I am filled with gratitude. Gratitude for the intensive conversations that developed in this exceptional situation, gratitude that I was able to have such an intimate experience in a foreign culture.

In the last terminal phase people are often too weak to paint. It is then possible to paint for them. Together you can look at the colours and perhaps talk about what is there, and what tries to come through. Maybe a broad landscape takes form in tender, pastel-like colours, or perhaps only colour moods.

Why are these light pastel-like tints important, and why are no strong, bright colours used in this terminal phase? In my experience with dying people, soft, tender colours speak strongly to them. In this phase every impression is 'impressive'. Who is not familiar with an inner timidity to enter the room of a sick or dying person out of fear to disturb them? Dying people have unsurpassed openness for their surroundings, for sound, smells, taste, voices, atmosphere. Their senses are oversensitive; all impressions and moods are perceived most intensely.

In this situation the art therapist must be careful with colours and colour impressions. Colours are connected with our feeling life. A dying person may experience colours much more intensively than we surmise. When colours are mild and soft, they can also easily show a perspective that is grand and light. Perhaps the spaces that are painted evoke memories, or it may be that a light space evokes a mood of infinite, grand openness, and that a longing grows in the soul for wide, light spaces.

Years ago I was asked to accompany a man who was in the very last terminal phase. He was bedridden and did not have the strength to do anything anymore. In addition to the conversations I had with him, he and I looked together at colours, and I painted for him. I stretched watercolour paper on a wooden board, and I started a simple veil painting. I had arranged the pillows on the bed in such a way that the man had a good view of the paper. Layer after layer I painted blue, yellow and red on the paper. Twenty to thirty minutes was enough for him, and this I did a few times per week. The intensive observation of the colours was clearly good for him; he visibly enjoyed the slowly growing painting.

One day I was working in this way together with him again. We looked at the broad, grand landscape that was slowly taking form on the paper. At a certain moment he asked me to step back a bit from the painting so that he could see it even better. I stepped back, and he looked and looked… Then he asked me to step back some more. His eyes were wide open – it seemed as if he was seeing more and more. Another step back, and another one, until I had my back against the wall.

Brightness and openness shone around him; radiantly his eyes were focused on the painting… Then he closed them and fell into a coma from which he never woke up. A few days later he died.

It will always remain a question as to what was happening in him in those last few minutes, but it is clear to me that the painting formed a bridge, as it were, to another world.

As the terminal phase progresses, we can distinctly observe that the circle of sense impressions becomes ever larger and more intense. The social circle, however, becomes ever smaller. There is less and less desire for contacts with the outside world, and interest in the outer world diminishes.

In this last phase of life we can sometimes witness how the power of discriminating between the essential and the non-essential becomes very clear and sharp. Intensive conversations with family and friends sometimes take place, in which inner connections unmistakably come to the fore. Problems in relationships that have been lingering for years may be expressed and dealt with. The themes discussed tend to relate to the inner life, the way destiny weaves between people. This inner process is a quiet, subtle phase, one of reflection in which enormous changes can still be achieved.

The inner attitude of the therapist who accompanies all this is, of course, of great importance. An inner space needs to be created for that which is inevitably coming. In these intensive moments, space and silence are important qualities. Artistic therapy or accompaniment here demands a constant sensing and probing to find the corresponding range of colours. There is no rule of thumb, because every human being goes through their own unique process to come to the end of their life on earth.

Veil painting

Using highly diluted water colours, veils are applied onto watercolour paper stretched onto a hard board. Initially the veils are so subtle you can hardly see them. Once a number of layers of paint have been applied over each other the colour becomes deeper and more intense. Because the composition in colour and form changes all the time during the work, it is a constant challenge in this type of painting as to what the next step will be. A unique feature of veil painting is ceaseless metamorphosis – one form dissolves into another. The work continuously changes in form and colour.

Connecting and letting go, courage and holding back, confidence in the process, playing and purposeful work alternate. Because of the variety of potential in the composition, decisions eventually become necessary as to the final direction. The growing dialogue between colour and form eventually 'invites' a definitive composition.

13

EXTERNAL THERAPY

Pauli van Engelen and Toke Bezuijen

Care in the last phase of life encompasses more than just medical and physical nursing. Actually, that is also true for all service and care. But in this last phase it is particularly desirable if we want to assist people in their longing for well-being and in their desire to conclude life in an emotionally and spiritually worthy manner.

Care with heart and soul

When we provide care in this sense, we enter into an especially close and involved relationship with the patient and their loved ones, a relationship that expresses patience, closeness and empathy, in which it becomes possible to sense or anticipate the wishes of the patient, even before they voice them. Care with heart and soul can give the patient an experience of healing – healing in the sense of well-being, a feeling of being complete, of being carried. A prerequisite for this is that we feel in our deepest essential being that we are equals.

When we care for the body, we at the same time touch the spiritual of the human being. Conversely, a good, open conversation can have a direct effect on a sense of physical well-being. All aspects of a bodily, psychological, relational and spiritual nature play a role in caregiving, for the human being is a holistic whole. This is true for the ill or dying person and their loved ones, but no less for professional caregivers.

Whether you are a nurse, caregiver or active friend or relative, the most intimate experience is always the loving care of the body as the sheath of the soul and spirit. Frequently the body is suffering from much discomfort, such as pain or cramps, stiffness, shortness of breath, cold or warmth (fever), dryness or dampness (perspiration).

To use Francis of Assisi's metaphor, our body, 'Brother Ass,' has enabled us throughout our life, from baby to old age, to gain profound experiences. But then the day comes when we are done with Brother Ass and have to let the spirit go its own way. Nurses and caregivers are in a unique position to observe this with respect. Their caring love for the suffering human being comes to expression in their manner of touching, of making contact with the hands, full of attention and at the same time competent, gentle and sure.

Seriously ill and dying people experience much at a very basic level; they sense our intentions bodily, non-verbally. When they are touched lovingly they will feel treated with respect; then they can relax and breathe more deeply, with the result that their pain and fear diminish.

In caregiving there always has to be the question: am I doing it in the way the person would like it? A bath with relaxing oil? Or a shower? Washing in the bed with delicate bath milk? Brushing the teeth, shaving, washing hair? What can the person still handle, and at what point is it too much? Washing is usually still possible, for instance, with lavender for relaxation and letting go, rosemary for refreshment or if more alertness is desired, or pine needles to relieve tightness in the chest. The dose can be adjusted to the scent the patient can still bear.

Of course there are many specific points that need attention, such as pain, wound care, bedsores, food and drink, constipation (often because of the use of morphine) or diarrhea, incontinence, shortness of breath, and so on. They deserve extreme care.

My seven-year-old daughter Lois was terribly ill for exactly nine months. When she was treated with chemo it became even worse. It was pitiful to watch. But somehow she remained very light and strong. At the time we saw an anthroposophic doctor who referred us to a nurse for external therapies. The nurse used many common plants and it always smelled so nice in Lois's little room, although the scents were not too strong, for Lois was very sensitive to smells. She liked to get a bath with scented oils once a week, and those were always her best days.

Later I was taught to give her a scented oil wrap on her abdomen, and I so much liked doing that. Even my husband could do something; every evening after her prayers he rubbed her feet, and usually she then fell into a blissful sleep. When we didn't rub her feet, she could not fall asleep easily. Toward the end, these treatments became shorter, but their effect seemed to be more intense.

In the meantime we had come to know the nurse very well and had a wonderful connection with her. Every time she knew how to help Lois with some little thing that made her feel better and relaxed her. In the end she did not need morphine at all; she died like a little angel in our arms.

External therapies

External therapies are applications such as wraps and compresses, special therapeutic baths and gentle rhythmical rubs. With all of these, healing substances are offered to the skin. The exceptional aspect of this is that in this way the more delicate senses of the skin are stimulated. After the treatment the patient is always swaddled in a flannel sheet and a woollen blanket (the 'packing'), in which they rest.

What makes these rhythmical rubs and baths unique is the combination of a healing plant, the quality of the hand or the water, rhythm, packing and subsequent rest. This generates a remarkable healing effect on the general feeling of well-being, while it stimulates the self-regulating functions of the organism. In all patients, their breathing becomes deeper, pain and fear diminish, and their sleep improves. Such treatments bring warmth, rest, relaxation and surrender.

A seriously ill young man of 29 years, whose death was near, received a complete body rub with rose oil once a week. Later the scent was no longer tolerated and a different essential oil was chosen. He often felt cold, but every time after the treatment he became warmer and felt more calm and cared for. Initially he had wanted euthanasia so as to be no burden to others, but after a number of these treatments that wish evaporated. He said that he could better bear the pain that was still there, and he became more and more relaxed. He felt strengthened on his path toward surrender and was able to say: 'I am very sad, but it is the way it is.'

The rhythmical rubs were followed by regular rubs of the heart region with rose-lavender-gold ointment; this helped him feel recognised in his grief. The treatments helped make the end of his life more peaceful.

– Evelien

Plants from Mother Earth

For these treatments we principally use natural products. These are produced with great care and attention, beginning with the growth and care of the plants. These are cultivated without poison, fertiliser, pesticides or artificial light. They get the time to grow by their own forces, build resistance, bloom and build up their own healing substances. Most of them are organic or biodynamic. In their cultivation the earth is not overtaxed but is meticulously nourished and cared for. You can tell by the greater fertility of the earth, the high quality of the medicinal plants, and ultimately in the quality of the products themselves.

There are many ways in which these products may be effectively applied. It is therefore important to remember that external therapy is a specialty. Do not just start doing something, but consult a external therapist.

For specific complaints several different medicinal effects of plants may be used. For instance, enemas against constipation may be made from chamomile tea; a cumin or fennel wrap may help against cramps or gas; lemon juice or bitter tea for nausea; self-healing of ascites can be stimulated by a quark or horsetail wrap; wounds can be cared for with herbal ointments such as marigold (calendula). In case of fever, the face, hands and feet may be cooled with peppermint tea. A beeswax compress, a thyme wrap or a lavender oil chest compress may relieve shortness of breath; and cramp can be relieved by rubbing the feet with lavender oil. Weakness may be relieved with a blackthorn rub. A heart rub with rose oil or gold ointment provides support in many different situations.

People who are seriously ill often feel cold, sometimes both cold and sweaty at the same time. A sheepskin and hot water bottles or little bags with warmed cherry stones (pits) may then be of help. If there is a lot of fear, a rubbing of the hands may be effective. Unrest may be relieved by putting a lavender oil compress on the chest, or a heart compress of gold, lavender and rose ointment.

In her last few days my mother was very restless, and although I often sat with her and held her hand, she kept giving me confused looks, and muttered and fiddled restlessly with the blankets. We had never been very physical together and didn't hug each other much and, to be honest, I didn't know whether that was called for now.

One day I happened to tell one of my art students about it; she was a nurse and asked me how my mother was doing. She suggested that I buy some lavender oil and, with warm hands, gently rub my mother's back with it while she was lying on her side. Afterwards I should sprinkle a little warm oil on a cloth and lay it on her chest on the heart. She also advised me to put a bag with warm cherry stones at her feet.

It was so moving to be able to do this. And really, she became quiet, and gently pinched my cheek. It reminded me of how she had cared for me as a baby; it felt so good and warm.

In the subsequent days I did it twice a day, and the night nurse also did it once. It quite relaxed her, and on the third night she passed peacefully away.
– *Anneke*

My husband could not let go; it was as if he was caught somewhere and, although he had said goodbye to all his loved ones, and everything seemed right, he was unable to cross the threshold. We did not know what was the matter. Then a sister-in-law who was a nurse, began to rub his feet very softly and quietly. The rhythm of this action, in which breathing in and breathing out were constantly visible, and the warm and loving touch with the copper ointment brought so much relaxation. It was as if it was saying: it is good, just feel it, it is good, you were a good man, it was good. It was like the memory of each year of his life every time her hands moved round again. It took at least ten minutes, and then he became so quiet, as if he was only then able to let himself go, as if he was gathered up by light.
– *Marja*

Also in mourning, external therapies may be helpful in carrying this very difficult process.

III

DEATH IS APPROACHING

At night in the desert,
Heaven so close,
Silence around me,
The earth sleeps,
The heavens watch,
The stars surround me,
So palpable, so near.

Memory rises in me
Of the world of old
For which I long,
What I miss is redeemed,
Heaven is not out there
But here surrounding me.

Renée Zeylmans

14

THE PHYSIOLOGY OF DYING

Paul Schmitz, MD

When we are going to die, the life processes let go of our body. The best way to study this is in the phenomenon of a slow death. We can then witness how the various members of our being cease to work.

At first the dying person can no longer stand up, or even sit up straight. The vertical position, the reflection of the I of the human being, is exchanged for a horizontal one. The warmth organisation, in which our humanity, the I, works in the physical, is less and less able to maintain itself. This means that temperature control in the person's immediate surroundings becomes more important, especially when they are being washed.

Changes also occur in the soul body. It gradually loses its ability to move the body; its connection with the body becomes looser. The senses become more acute; the reaction to sense impressions becomes more sensitive (see also Chapter 9).

The slow letting go of the ether or life body can be observed in the disappearance of thirst. When the life body is working very strongly, such as in a baby, the need for liquid (in proportion to body weight) is enormous. The dying person, however, often just needs to have the lips moistened, and hardly drinks at all.

Body-free experiences may also occur as the life body is loosening itself from the physical body, such as perceiving spiritual beings or people who have died. If such experiences are not recognised by the dying person, they may cause anxiety. Those around may easily interpret them as confusion or hallucinations.

As the life body continues to weaken, the circulation slows down, bedsores develop sooner, and moisture in the breath makes it audible. This rasping may be disturbing for bystanders, because they might think the person is suffocating, but in fact it is caused by superficial moisture in the throat.

The breath during dying

The breath is an important phenomenon during the dying process. Caregivers who have often been present during the dying process are able to follow its progress by the changes in the breath. In normal daily life we mostly don't notice our breathing. When we exert ourselves, the frequency and depth of our breathing increase; when we go to sleep, they decrease. Our breathing shows us how we connect with our physical body. Breathing in is always becoming a little more awake, while breathing out is falling asleep a little. We can notice it when we go to sleep, for then the emphasis falls more on breathing out. People who have difficulty breathing out, for instance due to a narrowing of the airways, often have problems falling asleep.

In the dying process it may sometimes take quite a while before the next in-breath is taken; we might even have the impression that there won't be another in-breath. But then several quick in-breaths follow, a long out-breath and... silence. This pattern, called Cheyne-Stokes respiration, is often present during a period in the dying process. There may also be periods when the dying person seems to be exerting themselves, shown in quick breathing, at first also quite deep, which then becomes more superficial. It is as if the whole body is asking to be inhabited again before it can be definitively released.*

A similar phenomenon also takes place with warmth; the body has

---

*A breathing pattern named after John Cheyne and William Stokes, the first scientists to describe it in the nineteenth century. The pattern consists of a long pause (apnea) followed by a phase of relatively quick breaths. It may occur in dying people, in heart failure, altitude sickness, and use of morphine.

to be warm from top to toe for the person to be able to die in peace (or simply to fall asleep). Cold feet often cause unrest, which disappears when they become, or are made, warm again (see also Chapter 13).

Consciousness during dying

The degree of consciousness with which people live through the dying process is individually very different. Sometimes people sleep a lot or are not really 'present,' sometimes they alternate sleeping with being genuinely awake. We often see that consciousness moves with the breathing pattern. This can most clearly be witnessed in Cheyne-Stokes respiration. In the quick in-breathing phase people are often present, whereas in the quiet out-breathing phase they fall asleep.

Pain could be viewed as enhanced consciousness. It is an unpleasant sensation, but (light) pain can also keep someone awake when the person has a tendency to lose consciousness. Strong painkillers may subdue consciousness, so that the dying person no longer has any awareness of the outer or their inner world. Except in cases of diseases that are specifically painful, dying in itself is not painful. But waking up repeatedly may also come with a kind of feeling of pain. Different individuals will deal with this in very different ways. It is important to understand how this works, because otherwise fear, not wisdom, will govern.

A final revival

An important phenomenon that I want to mention is pre-terminal revival, which regularly occurs in the last three days before death. It then seems as if any illness no longer matters, pain often becomes less, painkillers can be diminished or stopped. In people with dementia you sometimes see a revival of consciousness. I once experienced that a woman with dementia, who had not spoken for at least a year, started speaking again just before she died. Recognition of this revival is important for the way we assist the loved ones, in our approach to what is happening, and in order to realise that the last phase has begun (see also Chapter 17).

The dynamics of life

Most of the phenomena described in this book have been witnessed when the dying process takes between a few hours and many days. There are also people who die suddenly, or in their sleep. Looking back you can often say that someone 'did' their dying the same way in which they lived, especially from the point of view of the dynamics of their life or temperament. Of course the illness that carries a person to their death also has a big influence. In this aspect also, we can look at the dynamics to try and recognise how this illness fits into the life of the person who is dying of it.

15

EUTHANASIA

He who fears death either fears the loss of
sensation or a different kind of sensation.
But if you have no sensation, you will not feel
any harm, and if you acquire another form
of sensation you will be a different kind of
living being and you will not cease to live.

Marcus Aurelius, The Thoughts, *viii.58*

Fear of suffering

Fear of suffering, pain, loneliness – we all know what it is. Is there anyone who is not troubled by these? It is crystal clear that when we feel enveloped in safety, love and unconditional support and closeness, the question of euthanasia moves into the background. But also the question of the meaning of the painful process of dying plays a role.

If you believe that death is the end of everything, the question of prematurely ending one's life is, in my opinion, completely acceptable. After all, anything that has no perspective is unbearable.

> I have lived my life; I no longer have a future. I am ready for it.
> (An eighty-year-old man)

Is wisdom of life perhaps also wisdom of death? And is a perspective reaching across death maybe future expectation?

When my father died I had a strong feeling that I was in the
same realm as at the birth of my children. Just like at that time,
a portal opened.

– *Iona*

Perspective of a new life

In reality, preparation for the end of life pervades our entire life in a
hidden way. If we learn to face this underlying fear, perhaps we can
then transform it into more conscious life. Anything for which we do
not prepare ourselves – in other words, to which we do not develop a
relationship – may lead to a black hole.

Does an intention to commit euthanasia, when the time comes,
equate to a preparation for death? Such an intention could take such
possession of us in the terminal phase that we are more occupied with
the moment of the liberating injection than with our actual dying and
taking leave of our loved ones. And if, on top of this, we have a physician
for whom this is not a self-evident matter, and who is not inwardly
'ready' for it, an atmosphere of tension may develop. That is not a good
thing for the mourning process of the family. But if the intention to
proceed with euthanasia is a conscious, well-considered, inner decision,
it may very well take place in peace and harmony.

> My husband, Rob, died on December 10, 2004. He had lung
> cancer with metastasis into the head. Rob died surrounded by
> us – four daughters, two sons-in-law and our granddaughter of
> seven weeks – by means of euthanasia.
>
> Although it went exactly as the doctor had told us, for me
> it went much too fast. Rob's last words were: 'Darling, make
> something of life.' I said the text that would be printed on the
> announcement of his death: 'On wings of love the soul shall go
> home.'
>
> I felt broken and uprooted, as if torn asunder from each

other. Rob was so happy that he could go, his eyes were shining as if he was going to the greatest party. That day it was so still and quiet outside, as though a piece of heaven had come to earth. We were whispering and felt that a very special human being was going on a journey.

I have to think of bearing a child, of the delivery. This may often be a painful process, but one with perspective. In the end, the reward is the new life. And that is why it is bearable, for the father also.

If we have the perspective that our struggle with death is eventually the way to the light, our release from the stifling, sick body, we may perhaps find it less difficult to go through.

I had had anesthesia against the pain of the delivery, but when it then happened, I had such a strange, unreal feeling. Had I missed something?
– *A mother*

In cases of Caesarean birth that is also a frequently reported feeling. But also with euthanasia: 'It went so quickly.'

My colleagues and I feel that there is a different atmosphere around a person after euthanasia has taken place. It disturbs us; it is as if someone did not really die.
– *A nurse*

Self-determination

We live in a time of self-determination. An appeal is made to the I of the human being. We realise that it is important to take personal responsibility for our deeds. The other side of the coin is that we have to respect the decisions of our fellow humans.

Another name for self-determination is *salutogenesis*. This word consists of the Latin word *salus* (health) and the Greek word *genesis* (origin). Salutogenesis therefore has to do with the origin of health. The salutogenic principle is the capacity of the human being to deal with the foreign, with conflicts and, in doing so, to become stronger. We learn to recognise and push the boundaries of what we can physically and psychically bear. How do I learn to deal with all life situations and be flexible inwardly and outwardly? How do I develop a stable character?

In this context, even dying can become a last, meaningful growth phase. Whatever we then decide, whether or not we commit euthanasia, our eventual decision will be well-considered, so that we die the way we have lived.

> On the day when death will knock at thy door what wilt thou offer him?
>
> Oh, I will set before my guest the full vessel of my life – I will never let him go with empty hands.
>
> – *Rabindranath Tagore*, Gitanjali: Songs of Offering

Contemplation: O God!

God did not remove Himself from me,
But I removed myself from Him.

Blaise Pascal (1623–62)

As a child I always knew: God is love. Later I wrote it with an equal sign: God = love. In the course of my life this thought deepened. I feel that it has continued to infinitely deepen. It is like a 'life sentence'.

How often do we hear when some calamity happens: 'If there were a God, He would not let this happen.' And yet, we often exclaim 'O God' when we are frightened. Do we actually understand anything about God? Or do we all have our own private idea of God that he has to satisfy?

Pondering this I found something by the Jewish philosopher Hans Jonas (1903–93) that struck me.

Hans Jonas's mother perished in the gas chambers of Auschwitz. For him, a devout Jew, this was incomprehensible, for according to Jewish tradition God works in history, he works on and in history, and accompanies humanity in the historical process. God is experienced in history and does not punish the righteous.

After what happened in Auschwitz Jonas could only wonder: 'Where was God at the time of Auschwitz? Did he turn away from humanity and leave it in the lurch? Did he never exist? Or did God change his relationship with humanity? Did God develop his relationship with humanity further in the course of its evolution?'

With such questions Jonas arrived at an evolutionary concept of God, as he described in *The Concept of God after Auschwitz*. There he poses the question: Can God continue to be omnipotent and wise if it was possible for the Holocaust to take place?

He concludes that God can no longer be omnipotent and wise in relation to human beings; otherwise the Holocaust could never have happened. God has shared his omnipotence and wisdom with human beings. In so doing he gave them the freedom to choose the good, but also gave them the potential to err and to make the worst kinds of decisions. They must now know themselves what to do. They are themselves responsible for their deeds, not God.

Jonas discovered the middle realm as that of the truly human. It is the realm of the heart, conscience and love, which lets itself be united with the freedom of human beings and their autonomous insight. Only in this realm is a stable relationship between the human being and God possible, even from the very first days of creation to today.

Knowledge and power may be abused. They serve human beings to develop their capacities and consciousness of self. But love exists. It characterises the eternal essential core of human beings, with which God remains connected, also in Auschwitz. God is love. This God was able to be present in Auschwitz and give assistance to the people in the gas chambers. This concept of God after Auschwitz saved Jonas's view of God. But this concept of God is at the same time the most powerful salutogenic principle, the principle of the human spirit itself. It mobilises all sources of resistance that live in human beings. It answers the question: What enables me to resist physical, psychic and spiritual attacks to preserve my own health?

16

FASTING UNTIL DEATH

Fasting is renouncing eating and drinking. In a process of dying it is the most natural thing. At a certain moment the dying person will cease to eat and drink because the body no longer asks for it. However, fasting does not always happen in the terminal phase of life. Anyone, whether ill or not, may decide to fast. They then stop eating and drinking until death follows.

When we accompany a terminally ill person we may encounter such a conscious desire to fast, even if from a physical point of view it surprises us. The patient has the intention to shorten the dying process in this way. If we want to be a devoted companion we will do well to ask ourselves from what feelings and thoughts this wish proceeds, as described in the following.

By definition, a conscious decision to stop eating and drinking until death takes place in conversation with partner and family, with the explicit goal of causing or accelerating the moment of passing. The following information was taken from the psychiatrist Boudewijn Chabot's doctoral thesis *Auto-Euthanasia* of 2007.

In most cases eating is stopped first, followed by a gradual decrease in drinking. The feeling of hunger disappears after a few days. Clarity of consciousness is usually not impaired. The average time to death is ten days. If the person continues to drink, the process may sometimes last ninety days. Although there is documentation of a few painful deaths, the process usually proceeds well. In 70 percent of the cases studied, the family spoke of a dignified way of dying during which the person had lucid and pain-free moments to the last day.

The average age of people who choose to die in this way is 74 years. (People younger than 60 most often choose sleeping pills.) It is often said by the family of these people that they had a strong will. This way of dying confirms this, because the person is in complete control from beginning to end. One can begin it, but also stop it after some time.

Recent data shows that this is not something done by just a few people. According to the most conservative estimates, conscious fasting to death occurs thousands of times each year. It has been practised since the beginning of humanity. It has been described in antiquity, and research has shown that the Cathars in the Middle Ages were quite familiar with it, and in some cultures, including parts of India, it is highly respectable, because fasting to death there is viewed as a victory of the inner self over the body. It frees individual karma.

Conscious fasting until death by definition takes place in conversation with partner and family – Chabot emphasises this time and again. Death is then not the consequence of a deed, but of not doing something. In most cases a week passes between the beginning of fasting and death.

In my experience we can speak of an inner drama in fasting to death. Chabot points out that the people who want to end their life often do not want to die at all. On the contrary! They want to live, but without unbearable burdens. Chabot says that when, as a physician, he speaks with someone with an explicit wish to die, he looks for 'unfulfilled hankerings and hidden fear in the other.'

– *Marcel Seelen, in* Motief, *March 2008*

17

THE DOUBLE: MY SHADOW

The double personifies the shadow side of the human I, the emotions such as anxieties, hatred and jealousy that mostly live unconsciously in our soul. Our less attractive desires and passions, which we prefer to suppress because we don't know how to handle them, also belong to the domain of the double.

Unconsciously we often project these feelings and desires onto our fellow human beings. That which irritates us in others often has to do with our own shortcomings. This is an observation we have to face honestly time after time. 'Love your neighbour as yourself' (Mt 22:39). Perhaps we can only love ourselves if we first face the double in us honestly and lovingly.

The temple of Apollo the Greeks built in Delphi long ago had an inscription that even today has not lost its significance: 'Man, know yourself.'

When the moment of dying approaches

When you are told that your life is soon going to end, you may come into an intense confrontation with your shadow side. There is no more 'later,' at any rate, not on earth. In the very last phase of our life the definitive unmasking takes place. We wonder: 'Who am I? Who did I want to be? What is the meaning of life?' Our illusions melt away like snow in the sun. But the warmth of the sun that comes from the spiritual, supersensible world is a warmth full of love, which does not scorch us, but at all times envelops us in eternal, unconditional love. It accepts us completely as we are: the immortal core of our being, our higher I, our individuality, stripped of our shadow side which, by the way, does not come with us across the threshold.

> As a butterfly drawn by the sun
> Rises from its cocoon,
> My soul is freed from its earthly weight,
> And rises to the eternal light.

When we are with a dying person who is in the very last phase, it is of great importance that we are aware of what may take place when the double leaves them shortly before their passing. The double withdraws so that the human being may go through death. Usually this happens a few days before the person dies. It may be vehement, but it may also be experienced in silence by the dying person. Someone once said: 'Last night I met my dark double; that was not pleasant.' Three days later this person died.

The way this event expresses itself may be shocking and incomprehensible to the family. They had not known the person in that way. A modest woman, a patient who did not ask for much attention, sat straight up in her bed a few days before her death in a hospital and started ordering the nurses around like a general. Nothing was good; she was in a furious rage. This lasted a few hours; then it was over and she was able to die.

I was once present with a father who died at home and suddenly began yelling at his daughter and reproaching her for all kinds of things. When it was over he could hardly remember it. It did take some convincing to reconcile the daughter with her father again, but fortunately we were able to explain it to her and she understood. But I have also witnessed that the dying person became conscious of it after the fact and did not recognise themselves in it; that was extremely painful. It can destroy a relationship if one is not familiar with the underlying reason. Do not react to it; it is not meant personally. If you do react to it you feed the double who is loosening itself, and that makes the dying process more difficult. And if possible, do not give the person any medication and do not view it as a hallucination. Let it burn itself out.

Our own shadow side

In our mourning after the death of a loved one our own shadow side may show itself mercilessly. It may be like torment when we see what was of real importance in the relationship with the person who died. Through the identity crisis which mourning may cause in us we become able to distinguish the essential from the non-essential. Our sense of values changes.

During life we may be tempted to undervalue what we have, and put too much emphasis on what we don't have and so badly wish for. It hurts when we only realise what we had when we have to do without it. How often is 'love' not based on the expectation that the other will one day change the way we would wish? If the expectation is not realised, 'love' may disappear like snow in the sun. But whoever is no longer your friend, never was your friend. And when the white blanket of the snow has disappeared, everything under it becomes visible; and that may well be quite uncomfortable.

However, it is the sun which made this possible. The sun can scorch us with its heat and blind us with its light. But the spiritual sun can stream through us with its truth of self-knowledge, and thus show us undreamed of treasures.

For this reason mourning is more than grief alone. It is a new birth of the consciousness of our higher I, purified by grief and loneliness.

The double and I: I and the double

We may in our life have a feeling of discord, a kind of split, when we have good intentions but we end up doing the opposite of what we would like to do, such as words that seem to just roll out of our mouth and that we actually did not intend to say; or habit patterns we would like to break;

or a little voice that whispers something into our ear to which we would really not like to listen, but we still do it. What is it that is working there in me, and setting me on a wrong track? What is it that wants to mess things up all the time? When do I act out of my own sovereign will, and when does something act in me in which I am unfree?

We can get into a knot with our conscience. Our conscience sends us signals, calls on us to consider. What could we have known? What did we know? The Greek word for conscience (*syn-eidesis,* knowing together) indicates that there is an element in us that weighs and knows what we do and do not do. Maybe that is our higher I, which senses more accurately where the shoe pinches, what is acting up in our conscience. We then experience that we are like two human beings, our better self and our double.

What is unfree in us is what we would most like to push away, because it shows our less attractive side. But the more we try to repress our shadow side, the more it will manifest itself. This can bring us into inner conflict. It is as if we constantly lose the battle with our double. Only when we recognise our shadow side, if we can accept that part of ourselves, do we become able to face the inner conflict and deal with it, because then we have the weapon of insight. 'Man, know yourself!'

I was brought up with the Christian exhortation, love your neighbours. I chose great examples: Gandhi, Mother Theresa, Nelson Mandela. Thus I went into the world full of ideals to work in a slum in Africa, a project for the poor and homeless in Holland... I was always on the go for others.

Every time I got stuck, every time something went wrong that I had so badly wanted. Until I gradually began to realise, I am not Mother Theresa, I am not Gandhi, I am I. I must not follow their way, I must follow my way. And I took the first steps to begin doing what had been my favourite dream all my life, namely writing children's books. It felt terribly egoistic in the beginning! Doing only what I liked. I did not want to be an

egoist, I wanted to be a good human being, a good Christian!
It has been a huge battle, but now I know that what I do is not
egoistic. I follow my soul, and it is good this way.
– *Adriana*

Acceptance is a lifelong process that is not passive, but full of inner
activity. The double is not our enemy, even though it often feels like
that. If we can recognise it as part of ourselves, can look it in the eye, we
unmask it. Then the unseen enemy can become a teacher, and perhaps
we can bless the double and free it, as is expressed in the following
poem:

The Double

I have grown bent and crooked
With lifelong burdens
Forced on me.
There is no light, no face.
Only a voice
Takes hold of me:
I will not let you go.
I ask and seek,
I implore and curse.
I will not be a slave
Of my dark likeness.
Says he unmoved,
Without compassion:
I will not let you go.
And then he looks at me;
His gaze is murky
Like a cloudy sky
With its unending rain;
And suddenly,

As if the clouds tear open,
He calls to me:
I will not let you go,
Unless you bless me.
– *Bastiaan Baan*

Forgiving ourselves

In the physical world, the earthly, we are strongly focused on results. We may, however, feel confident that this is different in the spiritual world. Where there is no time, there is no final point, and therefore also no result. Ever and again we are allowed to try things again and do better. In fact, we die every day. We mourn things in which we failed. And we try to get up again! If we don't succeed right away, we need not be discouraged.

The higher I
I am not I,
I am the one
Who walks beside me
Without my seeing him,
Whom I do often visit
And often I forget.
He who is quiet when I speak,
Who gently forgives when I hate,
Who walks where I am not,
Who will remain when I die.
– *Juan Ramón Jiménez*

Who is this 'I' and who is it 'who walks beside me'?

Our real, true inner I is something we actually do not really bring with us into this physical world. We always leave it in the spiritual world. It was in the spiritual world before we came down into earthly existence. It is back in the spiritual world between our going to sleep and waking up. It always stays in the spiritual world. When we have our present-time conscious awareness as human beings during the day and call ourselves 'I', this word 'I' is a reference to something which does not exist in this physical world, though there is an image of it in this physical world.

– *Rudolf Steiner,* Initiation Science, *Sep 2, 1923, p. 55*

As human beings on earth we have no consciousness of what lives in our higher I. Because of this we make many false steps, but these teach us things, and isn't that what was intended? All the time, the higher I forgives the lower I its trespasses throughout our earthly life.

Father, forgive them, for they know not what they are doing.
– *Luke 23:34*

We also live in ignorance of the everlasting guidance the higher I gives us in collaboration with our guardian angel. We constantly try to reach up to the higher, eternal I and make a connection with it. If we do not succeed we have a feeling of tormenting impotence. But what in the outer world does not produce any visible result may in the world of the spirit be of decisive significance, albeit perhaps only in life after death.

Time and again we can experience, consciously or unconsciously, that we are but a part of reality. The path of schooling of daily life, nourished, for example, by meditation and prayer, offers us the possibility to re-establish this connection. The growth of self-knowledge, which helps us get to know our shadow side, will make us painfully conscious of the split in our being; on the one hand we strive to the divine in us, on the other hand there is the power of our desires and matter which shackle us to our little, lower I.

In this connection I am reminded of the biblical figure of Job. His material riches, the shining glitter that made him outwardly 'visible' to the people and friends around him were taken away from him. When he had nothing left, and even his family and friends turned away from him, the only thing he had left was his immortal core, Job himself. In this, the greatest struggle a human being can imagine, he entered into direct dialogue with God, and God awoke in him as a reality. God answered him, just as he answers everyone. But now came the struggle to understand God. Do I not like most to hear how good I am? And to receive the blessings I long for, irrespective of whether or not they are good for me?

A statement such as 'It is God's will' is perhaps no longer of this time. But in the depths of our suffering we can try to say: 'Your will be done. Your wisdom-filled love oversees my fate, my intention, my life destiny, so that my purified will may be transformed into wisdom-filled love after your image and likeness.'

This was achieved by Job, so that he could say:

My ears had heard of you but now my eye sees you.
– Job 42:5

This is what is left after everything else has been taken away from us. We stand like an onion of which layer after layer has been peeled off. We have taken off the coat of our selfish ego. Inevitably, some of the 'stuff' of the old coat will stick to us – we are human after all. Then a starry splendour descends from above and envelops us in a shining mantle. Never do we need to strive for perfection – that is the worst trap – for spiritual vanity may also lie in wait with its presumptuousness.

Our presence at death

It is death which dies,
Not life.
– Hazrat Inayat Khan

What a blessing for a dying person when their struggle and battle are recognised and we can truly walk beside them on part of their journey, thus living into the process. For we too experience the relativity of our existence. What are the achievements we take with us when we cross the threshold to the spiritual world? We realise that there is in fact no 'later,' only the here and now. And we then know that there are also other values than those of tangible material life; that what counts is to become aware of the value and meaning of life, the quality of life and the quality of death. The peeling of the onion then becomes the laying aside of all external things and attainments, until the highest quality of life is the only thing that remains. Then we no longer speak of humiliation, but of beauty and courage.

Whether the dying person will be able to show themselves thus, in all vulnerability, as they take off the earthly vestment, is perhaps the task of the bystanders. The result may then be that they do not need to observe themselves the way we look at them in their so-called humiliation because of our focus on the external, but that they are supported by our respect, our admiration for the struggle of letting go and taking leave, in which they go before us.

I am the last person to glorify dying. To observe and undergo the ageing and deterioration of the physical body can be quite uncomfortable. Every older person can confirm it; the mirror does not lie. We have to learn to live with that sight and grow into it; we have to learn to love the body. It has given us the possibility to manifest ourselves. Fortunately this coat does not become old or torn all at once; every wrinkle is a sign of having lived life. But the coat can be turned inside out. Have we regularly taken a look at the inside during our life, just as we use a mirror for the outside? Has the sound of our voice, the melody of our words changed? And the touch of our hands? How do we now walk our life destiny?

And then, at the very end, when we step across the threshold and let go of our earthly life, we leave the coat behind that we do not need anymore. The inside, the lining, with all its imperishable treasures we take with us. At last, we are able to *be*.

I look into utter darkness,
A light shines out,
Light that is alive.
Who is this light in the darkness?
It is my true and real I.
This does not enter into life on earth.
I am just an image of it.
But I shall find it again
When
With good will for the spirit
I shall have gone through the gate of death.
– *Rudolf Steiner,* Initiation Science, *Sep 2, 1923, p. 66*

18

THE MOMENT OF DYING

Ex Deo nascimur – out of God we are born
In Christo morimur – in Christ we die
Per Spiritum Sanctum reviviscimus –
through the Holy Spirit we regain life

Rosicrucian saying

The moment of someone dying is drawing near; we sense another dimension. We almost hold our breath, and step across the threshold with them. We hold back our own life forces. We may become very still, or we may be overwhelmed by feelings. We may also feel like two personalities, looking at each other, surprised. Much depends on the bearing and lucidity of the one who is dying, and whether or not there is acceptance, as well as on our reaction to this.

Two worlds come close together at the moment of dying, our earthly world 'broadens,' but the room is also filled with the presence of friends and family members who have died before us, and assist their loved ones, welcoming them as they are born into the spiritual world.

Where a spirit dies, a human being is born;
Where a human being dies, a spirit is born.
– *Novalis*

A holy silence

Suddenly, there is silence. It is a holy silence. Stay quietly with the one who just died; it is time well spent. You hand your loved one to the reception committee on the other side.

When we die we are taken across the boundary of life. The unity of the material body with the life body, the astral body and the I is broken. We rise up, as it were, out of our head. For the first time we receive a complete impression of our body as an object. We find our higher I-consciousness again. It is certainly not frightening. We leave our transience behind and move into eternity. We have a radiant awareness of birth and light. The Tibetan Buddhist Sogyal Rinpoche says about this that 'the divine being of radiant light shall appear to the newly dead in any form that they will recognise. Buddha for the Buddhist, Christ for the Christian, Muhammad for the Muslim.'

According to his explanation, this light is the great consciousness into which the consciousness of the one who died is taken up, the moment when liberation and enlightenment, can be realised. However, this can only take place after thorough preparation. This feeling of birth is beautifully described in the following:

> I was with my husband to the end. It was a difficult passing,
> he still wanted to live, remain with us, he kept resisting. That
> was painful. At the very last moment there was a gaze of
> astonishment; he saw something but could not express it, but
> I could read it in his face. It was as though he was illumined in
> warmth and colour. Whatever words I try to find for it don't
> come close to indicating what I observed with heart and soul.
> Then he went. I felt like a midwife toward the other world. I
> called my daughter who said: 'Mom, you sound so happy and
> relieved, but daddy just died!'
> – *Lili*

Take a little step into the 'timeless' where the dead person now dwells. Don't let the one who just died be taken away immediately. It is such a big transition if perhaps you have cared for someone for a long time, and then you suddenly stand in an empty room. Also prepare for this in a hospital, where people may want to act soon and clear the room.

> The moment my father died, his whole face lit up in an ecstatic
> smile that lasted for several seconds. His eyes opened wide
> and he gazed at a shining point in the distance. The shine also
> remained in his gaze after his passing. When after a short time
> the doctor came to officially confirm the death, he closed my
> father's eyes. I was very sorry he did that. I wish he would have
> asked us whether or not to do it.
> – Monique

> Place me like a seal over your heart,
> Like a seal on your arm;
> For love is as strong as death.
> – Song of Solomon 8:6

The Lord's Prayer

The Lord's Prayer is the central prayer of Christianity. It is an expression of archetypal wisdom. After it was once spoken by Christ on earth it has become a tremendous force which has been taken up into the cosmos forever. To penetrate into its profound significance we require ages and ages of human development. When we practise the prayer, when we let it work in us, it will reveal its power to us. It will strengthen our spiritual and earthly life. At any rate, this has been my experience in my life and work.

It is a prayer that contains no egoism. We do not ask for something we want from the Godhead, something that satisfies our own personal and often egoistic wishes, but we express ourselves in devotion and surrender: 'Thy will be done.' This actually strengthens our will, for Christ knows what each one of us really wills, stripped of all egoism and shortsightedness.

When the Lord's Prayer is spoken for a dying person, the words are directly taken in by the soul; the Christ in them is addressed. When we are present as bystanders, we experience perhaps that something is taking place that is greater than we are ourselves. When we say the prayer our soul reaches into the other. This makes it perceptible in the spiritual world.

> Our Father in the heavens,
> Hallowed be your name,
> Your kingdom come,
> Your will be done on earth as it is in heaven,
> Give us this day our daily bread
> And forgive us our trespasses,
> As we forgive those who trespass against us,
> And lead us not into temptation,
> But deliver us from evil,
> For yours is the kingdom, the power and the glory,
> For ever and ever.
>   Amen.

Rudolf Steiner said a version of the Lord's Prayer which he had developed out of his own spiritual insight. He said it aloud every night when he was alone in his bedroom. Various versions have become known. Below is the version Rudolf Steiner spoke with Ita Wegman when they worked on their medical book together in 1923–24.*

> Father, you who were, and are, and shall be in
>   our innermost being,
> May your name be glorified and exalted in us all.
> May your kingdom grow in our deeds and in the course
>   of our lives.
> May we do your will, as you, O Father, have laid it in our
>   innermost being.

*from Emmichoven, *Who was Ita Wegman*, Vol. I, p. 249.

The nourishment of the spirit, the bread of life,
You bestow upon us in abundance in all the changing
    conditions of our lives.
Let our compassion for others be compensation for
    the sins committed against our being.
Let not the tempter work in us beyond our power,
Since in your being, O Father, no temptation can exist.
For the tempter is but appearance and deception,
Away from which you, O Father, lead us through the light
    of your knowledge.
May your power and glory work in us throughout all
    ages of time.
    Amen.

IV

AFTER DEATH

Death is not extinguishing the
light; it is only putting out the lamp
because the dawn has come.
Rabindranath Tagore, The Heart of God

19

COINCIDENCE?

Coincidence is perhaps the pseudonym
of God when he does not want to sign.
Théophile Gautier La Croix de Berny (1811–72)

What a coincidence! Something fell into our lap. We often use the expression, for instance, when we accidentally run into someone, or when we are thinking of someone and the telephone rings because they are calling us, 'What a coincidence, I was just thinking of you.' Perhaps you open a book at random exactly at the page with the subject you were thinking of.

From my youth coincidences have always intrigued me. In some way or other I have always viewed them as indications that have something to tell us. If you become conscious of such things you gradually begin to understand the significance of what randomly seems to fall into your lap. You learn the 'language' of what comes to you, so that much of what happens in life becomes clear when you look back on it. You begin to see the golden thread in your life, with the result that you develop confidence in your destiny. My motto was always: 'What I don't see or know, need not be untrue.'

One thing I am sure of is that it has helped me bear the heavy loss of the sudden death of my husband. Not that my grief was any less, or that the awful, unjustified comfort of a friend was any easier to take: 'It had to be this way; it is your karma; life goes on.' Such consolation contributes nothing; it only makes you even more lonely and thrown back on yourself. These are things you may only say yourself, after a long time. You also don't need to overcome it all; you can only try to muster the courage and strength to get through it. My rock-solid conviction that coincidences do not exist has fortunately never been shaken, even in difficult situations.

Gertrud spoke of her husband, Peter, who had to say goodbye to life within a period of three months:

Peter was very sick. He knew he did not have long to live. He liked to organise things ahead of time, such as the way he wanted a funeral service in his favourite church, after an evening wake. But please not in a black hearse. Dan, a friend of his at work, had a great solution for this; he whispered in my ear one day that he had a beautiful white pickup truck in which he could transport the coffin. When I told Peter, he had to laugh. He thought it was a great idea, but he also said quite decisively: 'I can't do that. Then I would favour Dan over the other boys. But his truck would be great to transport the flowers.' (Peter wanted lots of flowers!) He thought it was a better idea to move the coffin in our new blue van. I thought that was an excellent plan.

When Peter had passed away Dan came by and said, 'The coffin doesn't fit in your van.' He was right. Well, then it had to be a black hearse after all. The evening wake, a wonderful gathering with much beautiful music, lovely words and a lot of tears, was on Monday evening. Peter stayed overnight in the church and the next day the funeral service was to be there too. After a very comforting service, many friends and relatives carried the flowers outside. In the sun they waited in a big circle for the hearse, while Peter was carried out by six good friends. The organ was playing beautifully, but... the hearse did not show up, it was stuck in traffic. The lady from the funeral home was very nervous. Well, we knew what to do: Peter clearly did not want to get into the black hearse. Dan was beaming. 'Get your truck, Dan,' I said. 'You can take Peter.'

You cannot imagine a prettier picture: a large group of waiting people, a shiny pick-up with open cargo area into which the white coffin was pushed and covered with flowers. I fetched our van for the rest of the flowers. The three of us, my son, daughter and I, followed the white truck to the cemetery. It was a sad but happy parade.

When we arrived at the cemetery hundreds of people were waiting there. They took the flowers and formed an honour guard along which Peter was carried to his grave by his friends. The sun was shining, children had white balloons, and after the Lord's Prayer we were the first to throw some soil on the coffin.

It may sound strange, but I have wonderful memories of this day, also of the gathering afterwards when we all raised our glasses in celebration of the life of this dear man. I have a distinct feeling that he had the reins firmly in his hands that day, and he saw to it that we would not just be sad. He was very much with us!

Butterflies

The butterfly is a universal symbol of the liberation of the spirit from the constraints of the body.

During the funeral we can become aware of many things if we have our eyes and ears open. We might note the weather, a rainbow, the sunrays, birdsong, and so on. It is remarkable how many stories there are of butterflies that appear at crucial moments. Perhaps it is no coincidence. In old mythologies butterflies were viewed as the souls of those who had died, and they were therefore left untouched.

During the Second World War the captives in the concentration camps of Buchenwald and Dachau had carved names, initials and drawings into the walls of the barracks. But also butterflies, lots and lots of butterflies. People often spontaneously tell me butterfly stories, even though they do not always know their meaning.

My neighbour, who is 81, told me once about an event after the death of her husband. The last seven years of his life she had taken care of him at home with the help of visiting nurses. During the funeral service a monarch butterfly (which is not common in that area) flew into the church. I don't think she had seen it, because one of the grandchildren had caught it and taken it outside, where it quickly flew away.

When she was visiting the grave with her daughter a few days later they wondered how the father/husband would be, and whether he would know that they were standing by his grave. Without words the daughter inwardly asked her father for a sign of life. When they looked up, right over the path the monarch was flying in their direction. He flew to them in an unusually straight line and perched on the trunk of a birch tree opposite the grave. The daughter told her mother the story of the butterfly in the church. They both knew that this animal of the resurrection brought them an answer.

– *Paul*

My father makes contact with me, his daughter, via a white eagle. In his younger years my father had been in the Dutch army in Indonesia. He didn't talk much about it, but he did go to the reunions of his unit to see his mates. An eagle figures in the emblem of his unit. I was familiar with this bird with its white head from early childhood. It was part of my father.

After my father's passing my mother and I went to visit my sister in America. My parents had also done that together a few times. My dad would then go fishing on a river with my brother-in-law. I went to 'their' spot along the river with my brother-in-law to look for a pretty stone to put on Dad's grave in Holland. The moment I saw a pretty stone an eagle flew over my head. I took that stone with me. My brother-in-law was astonished, as eagles never come there during that time of year.

He looked for his camera, but by the time he had found it the eagle had flown away.

Last summer I stayed with my sister again, for two delightful weeks. The moment of saying goodbye was always difficult; we both went about the house crying. I sat down in the garden for a moment. When I looked up I saw an eagle soaring round and round over the neighbourhood. I called my sister, we both knew the story, and said: 'It is good.' Then another eagle came and together they circled low over the house and garden. It all took about ten minutes. We had a warm, happy feeling.

Thank you, Dad. I am going back to Holland but my sister is staying in America with her husband and child.

Back home I participated in a community walk. I often did that with my dad. Afterwards I stopped by his grave and stood there deep in thought when there was suddenly a big raptor flying over my head. It came to greet me.

It is crystal clear to me: my dad tries to make contact with me in the form of an eagle.

– *Liesbeth*

A mother confided an experience to me:

We were in a vacation house in France and were having a lazy morning. When I got up and went to the kitchen I heard loud music. I saw our house friend sitting at the table outside with a cup of coffee, quietly enjoying the view of the lake. I wished her good morning and asked her whether she enjoyed the music, as it was the CD of our son who had died the year before. 'Yes,' she said, and asked whether my husband had turned on the music. I looked at her and said: 'I thought you had turned it on.' 'No,' she said, 'the music started as I was sitting here.'

I walked to the kitchen and then realised that my husband wasn't even up yet. Still I went to ask him, but he answered that no, he had not turned on the music. A mystery! When we had breakfast together we looked at each other and talked about the fact that none of us had turned on the music. It was the music that our son, who had died that day the year before, liked very much; and he also loved this spot in France.

Together we walked to the CD player and looked at it in surprise. We then realised that some time last year we were also in this house together and, of course, with our son. Are you letting us know that you are with us, on this spot where you felt so at home and so much liked to come? You certainly succeeded in making your presence known! We all agreed that this could be the only explanation.

Later that day we called our other son and told him the story. He was also surprised and amazed, and told us that he had played the same CD in his car at the same time.

An unforgettable experience for all of us that continues to amaze us. A signal from the other side, like: I am with you and will stay with you!

20

THE FUNERAL

'What is a rite?' asked the little prince.
'Those also are actions too often neglected,' said
the fox. 'They are what makes one day different
from other days, one hour from other hours.'

Saint-Exupéry, The Little Prince

Rites and customs give a sorely tried soul something to hold on to. The funeral is the final chord of a life. You may sometimes be aware – either in a kind of dreamy state or in clear consciousness – of the presence of the one who has died. If a life in a sick or disabled body was difficult, it may be granted us to 'see' the radiating freedom itself during a funeral.

During one of our courses in accompanying the dying and mourning, one of the participants told us what she saw during the funeral of a very good friend who had been seriously handicapped all his life. His shining figure, freed from the body, spread out, as it were, over the people gathered. She felt inexpressible blissfulness streaming out from him.

Of old, the rituals around all the events of dying, the wake, the funeral have had a connection with the spiritual world. Without that connection these are symbolic acts that have mostly to do with ourselves and with the here and now. If the funeral is an honestly ensouled interplay of respectful or sacramental acts, it may be intensely experienced. It can be a real support for the family, a connection between heaven and earth. It may make a big impression if one or more family members or close friends relate something of the course of the person's life. Perhaps that may bring about a recognition for those present as well as for the soul of the dead person: 'Yes, that was me. That is me.'

My brother died suddenly. The Second World War had left its mark on us. My brother once said to his wife, 'I put my feelings under lock and key; no one can get to them.'

And that was the way it was. His wife and children knew nothing about his youth; the first twenty-five years of his life were missing in their picture. I became aware of the fact that our childhood years, the care and loyalty he had shown for me as a small child, were the key to the real being of my brother, to the picture I wanted to keep of him.

I was the only one who had a complete picture of him. And now, after his passing, I had to tell people about our childhood years. In the privacy of his family this was not so difficult, but with the hundreds of people at his funeral it was really hard.

After the funeral many people came to me to thank me for the story about our childhood. 'That had always been a missing piece,' they said. Now they had seen who my brother really was.

Never had I experienced so clearly that the biography of every person is inseparably linked to the picture of them that people have in their heart. It gives you the possibility to be with the person in your thoughts. And for the survivors that is a great help. But isn't it also important for the one who died, how people on earth think of him or her?

– *Frederick*

The final resting place

Upon arrival at the grave you might choose to lower the coffin yourself. You might also choose to throw some dirt onto the coffin. This may be a good thing for children because it is so logical for them: when you bury someone, they should be under the earth! If they are anxious, it is often caused by our own fear of death. In case of cremation you might consider staying with the coffin until it goes to the furnace. If that is what you want to do it is good to arrange it ahead of time.

After the funeral you might want to take some of the flowers home to let them wilt there, for instance, in the garden.

Burial or cremation?

If the person who died made no decision as to whether they wanted to be buried or cremated, the family has to make the choice. In addition to practical things, you could consider the following aspects.

Whatever choice you make, it makes no difference to the one who has died. Rudolf Steiner was one who emphasised this. But he did suggest that for a small child who has not yet had an experience of the inner 'fire' in the course of their life, burial is perhaps preferable. A grave is also a good memorial for little brothers and sisters.

He also indicated that burial is preferable for a suicide. The soul might have a need for an orientation point, because the person who died had themselves determined the hour of death and might continue to feel a bond with the body for a period of time. These are just considerations; the choice may and will depend on each individual; people are unique.

When we bury our dead we return them to the elements of earth, water and air. When we cremate them we return them to the elements of air and fire and, if we scatter the ashes, also to the earth.

Contemplation: The number forty

The number forty has been on my mind for a long time. Why do we run into it so often? According to the Church Father St Augustine, the number forty signifies the earthly life of burdens, wanderings and expectations.

In the Bible the number forty plays a large role. For example, the Flood lasted forty days and forty nights, as did Moses's stay on Mount Sinai to receive the commandments (Ex. 24:18). After Jesus's baptism in the Jordan follow forty days of temptation in the desert. The wanderings of the Israelites lasted for forty years. The Sinai desert is not that big: symbol or reality? What does forty years indicate?

The Church has frequently used the number in constructing its calendar. Lent, from Ash Wednesday to Easter, lasts forty days; from Easter to Ascension is also forty days. During that time the Christ spirit permeates the earth with resurrection forces.

In our lives the number forty also plays a larger role than we perhaps realise. A pregnancy lasts about forty weeks from conception to birth. The spirit incarnates into a body. But after the birth it takes another forty days for the spirit to arrive into the body, to penetrate the physical with the soul. The baby then begins to develop a focused gaze and to smile consciously.

The same time span is still used for quarantine measures, which of old lasted forty days. The French word *quarante* means forty. It was the time that was deemed necessary to be purified of an infection. And then there is the saying: 'Life begins at forty.' Why? Perhaps because at that point the spiritual has matured and can be manifested.

In many cultures and religions, including the Jewish, Muslim, Catholic and Greek Orthodox religions, the fortieth day after death is considered as a day to remember the person who died; the first awakening is celebrated! The human being is born into the spiritual world, has 'landed.' We have already seen that we can observe the same phenomenon with a child that is born on earth: around the fortieth day we see their first real smile!

For a long time I have made a connection between forty days and certain events in our lives, for instance, after an illness, surgery, accident, emotional experience, and so on. It is my experience that we need this time for inner processing in order to, as we say, find the 'ground under our feet' again. Viewed in this light, it is a good idea to revive an old ritual that has become lost in our time, namely to say a verse or prayer for your beloved who has died, for forty days. This helps both him or her and yourself.

21

ACCOMPANYING THE DYING AND CHRISTIAN RITUAL

Bastiaan Baan

The greater the knowledge, the more reverential
it will become, for worship is the only possible
way to make contact with divine reality.

Frieling, Im Zeichen der Hoffnung, *p.106.*

Ritual is a way of making contact with the divine world that literally and figuratively speaks a very different language than the everyday ways we use to communicate with each other. This is one of the reasons why many people have difficulties with the idea of ritual, even though around the special high points and low points of human life there is a need for rituals of all kinds. We often look for a meaningful ceremony or ritual, and we increasingly tend to give it a form ourselves. For example, a funeral home recently advertised, 'It can be done in many different ways.' Just like in other areas of social life 'anything goes' seems to be the motto. As a result, accompanying the dying and the dead has become an intensely personal matter.

Irrespective of fashion, which sooner or later will come up with other novelties, in all times and in all cultures we find ritual forms through which people who are dying or who have died are accompanied. In a religious ceremony or ritual a connection is made between word and prayer on the one hand, and ritual substances on the other. A well-known example in Christian ritual is the use of bread and wine.

Not only the words and prayers, and not only the substances of bread and wine, but the connection between word and substance or element makes the ritual act complete, makes it into a sacrament. Thus literally sounds the formulation by Church Father Augustine, 'The word is added to the element, and it becomes a sacrament.'*

Of old there have existed seven Christian sacraments that work from birth (baptism) to death (last anointing). The substance used for baptism (long before Christianity already) is water. For the last anointing oil is used. But all kinds of ritual acts for after death, generally performed with substances such as incense and water, have also been known since antiquity. These were used in ritual acts for the dying and the dead, not only as 'last aid' on the way to dying, but also as 'first aid' in the life after death.

Ritual acts around dying have always had this significance, not only in Christianity, where the Resurrection is of decisive importance, but also in pre-Christian and other ritual acts, for instance, in the Egyptian and Tibetan Books of the Dead, which were read to the dead, together with ritual acts. Through these the dead person was helped to awaken to the spiritual world and to continue life in another form of existence.

In early Christianity the day of death was called *dies natalis,* day of birth, because the first Christians had the conviction that the dead person was born anew thanks to Christ who was risen from death. This belief was not just a teaching or conviction, but it was deeply 'lived' by the first Christians who were persecuted and killed for their belief. For the Romans, who fought Christianity in its early days, this was the most characteristic and unsettling aspect of the new faith: they had no fear of death.

This difference in the view of death is notably documented in two quotations which, in their contexts, represent two entirely different worlds. The Apostle Paul wrote out of deep conviction: 'I face death

* *(Accedit verbum ad elementum et fit sacramentum.) Tractates in the Gospel of John,* 80.3.

every day – yes, just as surely as I rejoice about you in Christ Jesus our Lord.' The Emperor Tiberius wrote in his despair almost the same as Paul but meant the opposite with his statement: 'May all the gods and goddesses destroy me more miserably than I feel myself to be daily perishing.'* For Paul death is the beginning of a new life; for Tiberius it is the absolute end.

In Christian religious services we find the frequent entreaty to be reborn in the spirit, an entreaty for which ritual substances give expression to a new life in another form of existence. Consecrated oil is an ancient means of accompanying someone across a threshold. Oil was used for the anointing of kings and priests. Both priest and king – even if each in very different ways – have the task to rise above the personal so they can serve a higher world. Similarly, a dying person is anointed with oil in order to cross the threshold of personal, earthy life and evolve into a supra-personal, spiritual form of existence.

In old rituals, water was sometimes called *aqua regenerationis,* water of regeneration. By pronouncing certain prayers over the water, it is consecrated. The earthly element of water thus becomes the carrier of spiritual powers, in this case, renewing, regenerating forces. The other sacramental substance that is used with the dead is incense. When incense goes up in smoke it becomes an eloquent symbolic expression of the transition of a visible to an invisible existence.

Like a golden thread the quintessence of the Christian faith runs through all the ritual acts around dying: 'He is risen.' Together with the dead person, the priest addresses Christ, who leads souls into the realm of the dead. In Christian rituals, Christ is often quoted – and here we have to hear the word 'cited' in both of its meanings. The words of Christ are repeated (as a citation), but in doing so we at the same time 'incite' his presence. That is the original significance of ritual acts. They do not stand alone, but priests 'serve at a sanctuary that is a copy and shadow of what is in heaven' (Heb 8:5).

---

* Tacitus, *Annals* VI, 6.

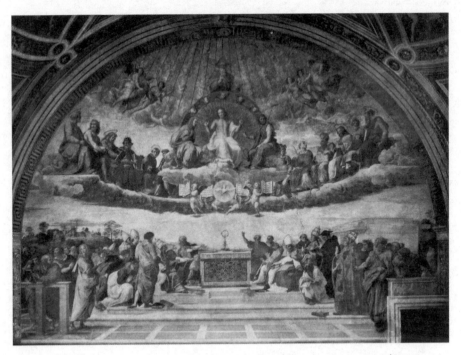

Ritual as 'a copy and shadow of what is in heaven' (Heb 8:5). Disputa *by Raphael (Vatican, Rome).*

Those who are able to behold what takes place in heaven through clairvoyant observation, will recognise that the earthly priestly service is complemented by the ritual that is celebrated at the same time in the spiritual world. The earthly and the heavenly acts, the visible and the invisible rituals, correspond with each other. Thus it literally sounds in the description of a funeral ritual in which, beside the earthly 'mirror image,' the spiritual 'archetypal image' is perceived.

Rudolf Steiner recognised in the funeral ritual of the Christian Community* no more and no less than a mirror image. It is a true mirror image, which is an earthly likeness of a spiritual reality. Concurrently

---

* The Christian Community, Movement for Religious Renewal, was founded in 1922 by a group of young theologians with the help of Rudolf Steiner. In this movement the seven sacraments are formulated and symbolized so that modern consciousness can follow them and inwardly co-celebrate them. Another expression of this renewal is that the Christian Community has no dogmas.

with the funeral ritual, in which we take leave of the person who died, the spiritual hierarchies, the angels, receive his or her soul and spirit in what Rudolf Steiner called a 'welcoming ritual.'

In this way, in a form of ritual that has been gleaned from the spiritual world, mirror image and reality, parting ritual and welcoming ritual, correspond with each other. The person who died receives assistance from two sides, from human beings and from angels, on their way into life after death.

At the end of Rudolf Steiner's description it becomes clear that what is important in a funeral ritual is not only the 'what' but also the 'how.' Not only the correct words, acts and substances determine the power and effectiveness of the ritual, but also the manner in which the words are spoken and the acts performed:

> If we celebrate a true ritual for the dead, a supersensible ritual
> is enacted simultaneously. The two work together. And if there
> is sanctity, truth and dignity in the prayers for the dead, then
> the prayers of the beings of the hierarchies in the supersensible
> world echo in the prayers for the dead and weave in them.
> – *Steiner*, Karmic Relationships, *Vol. II, June 27, 1924, pp. 237f*

In this text, Rudolf Steiner described the funeral ritual of the Christian Community, as it appears to clairvoyant observation. In the text of this ritual we hear two well-known motifs which we also find in older ritual forms. Thus the Latin Requiem describes the world of the dead in two oft repeated phrases:

> *Requiem aeternam dona eis Domine.*
> *Et lux perpetua luceat eis.*
> (Give them eternal rest, Lord. And let perpetual light shine
> upon them.)

The dead enter a world of rest and a world of light. In the funeral ritual of the Christian Community these two motifs return, now in connection with the way of soul and spirit after death:

> The soul walks in the calm of soul being.
> The spirit enters into the light of the spirit world.

Together with the first motif of the funeral ritual, in which is described that the material sheath is entrusted to the world of the elements, the classical trichotomy of body ('the mortal sheath'), soul and spirit comes to expression here – in which soul and spirit each experience a different reality in the world after death. The soul with all its 'movements' gradually comes to rest; the immortal spirit can disengage from body and soul, and enter into a world of light.

Thus the alpha and omega of the experience of death is expressed in eloquent words: death separates what was indissolubly linked throughout life. Body, soul and spirit are severed from each other, and each goes its own way.

What is really decisive for ritual reality, however, is not just that the right words and acts are celebrated by an ordained priest, but especially that the ritual is celebrated in a particular manner: 'And if there is sanctity, truth and dignity in the prayers for the dead, then the prayers of the beings of the hierarchies in the supersensible world echo in the prayers for the dead and weave in them.' Without sanctity, without truth and dignity, the words remain empty husks. In that case they lack the power to reach the one who died, let alone the hierarchies.

Thus it becomes understandable that especially the 'how' (in addition to the 'what' of the ritual act) is decisive for the presence of the spiritual world, which is being called on. The quality of reverence is reflected in a particularly impressive manner in the following experience:

> When on Sunday morning people participate in a service of
> worship, become inwardly quiet, listen to the organ and to
> the priest who reads the Gospel, a mood of reverence may

grow. That is an atmosphere the spiritual world loves. Thus it happened one Sunday that suddenly a spiritual being appeared, that was at first like a shadow. I could not quite make it out. Later this shadow-like being came more often. I did not ask what it could be, because I had already learned that the spiritual world does not like curious people and immediately withdraws from them.

Then came Holy Week, two years ago, and now I saw that the same figure I had seen a number of times was an angel. Suddenly he stood like a radiant figure beside the altar. He stayed there only for a moment. Then he hovered quickly and lightly, the arms crossed over the chest, in front of the first row and full of goodness looked the first person who sat there in the eye. Then he went to the next person. With this wondrous expression in the eyes he hovered from one person to the next and looked each one in the eye. In retrospect I realised that it can hardly have been more than three seconds, but it is possible to observe a person in a short time.

Then I had to think: but this is the angel of the congregation. No one else would be able to do this in the same way. And suddenly it was clear to me that this angel observed each of us individually. When he came to the second row, where I was sitting, I felt his eyes directly on my face. I can only say that it was a profoundly moving impression to sense, to know: this is the angel of the congregation who participates in us, as we also participate in this worship service.

I am certain that in every church of whatever denomination, where there is a mood of reverence, where the Gospels are really read, where politics are kept out and only what is Christian streams in, there is also an angel of the congregation who looks the people in the eye, hoping also to be observed by them.

– *Wegener,* Blick in eine andere Welt

Ritual for the dead is more than a 'travel guide for the hereafter,' in which life after death is described. When during life we have practised reverence in our efforts to make contact with the spiritual world, we will experience after death that the spiritual world will receive us in joy and give us wings.

22

MOURNING BY FRIENDS AND RELATIVES

For with much wisdom comes much sorrow;
The more knowledge, the more grief.

Ecclesiastes 1:18

If completely shut out from the outer world, you dwell in a space of intense pain. It is as if your body no longer belongs to you. And yet you minutely observe everything; your senses are strained to the limit in an unprecedented wakefulness, while at the same time you have a feeling that you do not truly inhabit your body. Your soul has withdrawn. Your limbs aren't really part of you anymore but they function automatically from memory. You are dwelling in a realm of soul pain; this pain has nothing to do with your body or your intellect. The soul has contracted into a realm without past or future. You have become estranged from the world you thought was reality, but now you know that it is merely a reflection of the reality of eternal, imperishable being. You are a spectator of yourself.

A path of initiation

This is actually a near-death experience, a path of initiation! Hurled out of your body by a tremendous shock, you land in a space that cannot be described in words. It creates a unique, timeless feeling that can only be recognised by people who have gone through it themselves.

This experience, this despair, this pain of intense grief, are caused by your love and intimate connection with the person of whom you had to take leave. It is like the pain of an amputation; not a sign of weakness, but of true connection. To love another being so deeply that you feel not only your own pain but also their pain of taking leave, is like going through the eye of the needle. But it is also the way to the light, the labour pains of being born on the other side. At the same time, you can also sense the joy of their deliverance.

> It takes courage to leave,
> It takes courage to remain.

Everything has its counterpart: joy and sorrow, light and darkness, day and night. The one is not more than the other. No, they make each other visible, they complement each other. In mourning, moods and feelings constantly vary. A painful moment, for example, may change into a moment of unprecedented joy, which the very pain enables you to feel.

Kahlil Gibran has a striking way of expressing it:

> Your joy is your sorrow unmasked.
> And the selfsame well from which your laughter rises
> Was oftentimes filled with your tears.
> How else can it be?
> The deeper that sorrow carves into your being,
> The more joy you can contain.
> ...
> Some of you say, 'Joy is greater than sorrow,'
> And others say, 'Nay, sorrow is the greater.'
> But I say unto you, they are inseparable.
> Together they come,
> And when one sits alone with you at your board,
> Remember that the other is asleep upon your bed.
> Verily, you are suspended like scales
> Between your sorrow and your joy.
> – *Kahlil Gibran*, The Prophet, *p. 35*

I regularly see clients who are desperate but, at the same time, do not dare or are unable to mourn, because they feel guilty for their grief. They do not want to burden the one who has died with their pain; they do not want to claim them, be egotistic. But do we really burden the dead with our grief? I don't think so. Someone who creates soul connections out of profound sorrow does something beneficial for the dead person.

If we would claim the dead we would indeed burden them, but in all the years of my therapeutic practice I have actually never experienced that someone really claimed a dead person. To claim is a hard, constant form of wanting to possess for ourselves. That is something completely different from the struggle of mourning, with all its moments of profound pain and loneliness, moments of appealing and imploring mingled with the hope and wish that the other is well. The one who died also wishes for clarity, also wants to confess, to face things, to forgive and be forgiven. Mourning is a dialogue.

In despair between two worlds

Your path of initiation is the process of dying along with the dead, being able to have a glimpse of the world of the dead. It is the crossing of a threshold. This may create a feeling of unreality, of living in two worlds. The unique aspect of it is that you don't actually lose your ability to function on the physical plane; in fact, you can be very lucid. You register everything, but you can't always react adequately, because your heart and soul are dwelling in another realm. But you do take everything in.

This is not a condition of shock, as conventional medicine wants to make us believe. That is a 'translation' for those who do not know the other side of truth. A half truth!

Let us always approach with respect the things we have not experienced ourselves and cannot explain. What we don't see or know need not be untrue. Your great love and compassion may from time to time transport your soul into the realm of your higher I; with your immortal core, your higher self, you can find a balance in despair between two worlds. You can metamorphose, grow past the suffering and thus develop capacities to make gifts to your fellow human beings.

Raising the cross in yourself – this is only possible if you have taken the cross of suffering into yourself, horizontally connected with humanity, vertically with the spiritual world.

Dying, mourning, comforting

It is a fact of life in the time in which we live that we feel cut off from the dead, that there is a here and a there. The separation may feel like a wall. Part of this are despair and pain, feeling cut off; but also moments of nearness, of connection with the dead transcending death. Out of this soul pain a close connection may grow in the course of many years.

Dying, mourning, comforting – three concepts that are indissolubly linked together and form part of the process we call life. But we can only truly understand each other on earth – and perhaps this is also true for our contacts with those who have died – if we are able to recognise the painful way of someone else, and we thus acknowledge it in its essential truth.

Loss

Can you describe pain
Of being severed
The emptiness inside
The confusion
In heart and head
The cold in my bones
The want?
Learning anew to walk
On a path never tried
Searching, groping

For a glimpse of light
A trail of tears
Softens the earth.
  – *Fieneke van Wees*

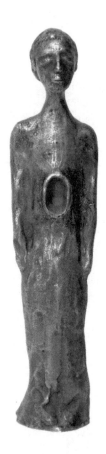

Simonette Beenders, bronze from the series, And the sea… it took you along.

23

ACROSS THE THRESHOLD OF DEATH

A shiver plays through the aspen,
The evening glow shrinks back
And all that was ineffable and far
Is ineffably near.

Gunnar Ekelöf (1907–68)

In my practice I am often asked the question, full of grief, 'Renée, where is the one whom I loved so much now?' A person dying may also ask us, 'Where am I going, what will happen to me?'

Through the ages every culture, every religion, has tried to find an answer to that question. From old books and wisdom we can form an imagination for ourselves of what is awaiting us across the threshold of death. But also stories from our own time told by people who have had a near-death experience give us a clue.

A different appearance

When we die we let go of our physical body and return to the spiritual world, the world from which we were born. Our personality shrouds itself in a different appearance, one that is not bound by time or distance.

> The trick, according to Chiang, was for Jonathan to stop seeing himself as trapped inside a limited body that had a forty-two inch wingspan and performance that could be plotted on a chart. The trick was to know that his true nature lived, as

perfect as an unwritten number, everywhere at once across
space and time.
– *Bach,* Jonathan Livingston Seagull, *pp. 59f*

After death we have to learn to do without our physical body. Because
it is no longer there we cannot gratify our passions, desires, needs and
longings anymore. Despite the fact that we no longer have our physical
body, all these forces, which made use of the body, are still actively
present, depending on the extent of our need of physical gratification.
The more we were able to detach from such physical needs on earth,
from passions and desires, the less difficult it will be to overcome our
longing for the old sheath, and the more comfortable we will be in our
new sheath in the spiritual world.

The review: a mighty symphony

When we die and we let go of our physical body, we pass the threshold
of the spiritual world. As the life body gradually loosens itself from the
physical body, memories are freed, and the impressive tableau of the
life we have led spreads out before us in all its fullness. We observe
every event in our life, not overwhelmed by subjective feelings of lust,
obsession, joy or sorrow, but objectively and in relation to the greater
whole. Herbert Hahn related the following about this:

[Rudolf Steiner] reminded us of how shortly after death the
soul sees its life moving past like a great panorama, in pictures
that show in swift succession every detail of the just completed
life. But the beauty of it is, Steiner continued, that this world
of pictures is at the same time filled with sounds, and can be
experienced musically. Like a mighty symphony the entire
cosmos streams toward these sonorous images and absorbs
them into itself. In the midst of this symphony the listening
soul, however, suddenly hears how one sound, one note, clearly

stands out in the abundance of all the other sounds. It is a unique experience; one hears the whole but still, this one separate tone, with its pristine sound, stands out against all others. And suddenly the soul arrives at a wondrous insight: without me the world symphony would not be complete.

Nothing during the entire life on earth – and hardly any other moment in life after death, Steiner added – can be compared in such complete bliss with the experience of the human being who, just freed of the yoke of earthly frailty, comes to know the great secret: I am an indissoluble part of the great totality of the world; without me the world symphony would not be perfect.

– *Hahn*, Wir erlebten Rudolf Steiner

After about three to three and a half days the family can see from the face of the person who died that the life forces have left the body. This also signifies the end of the life tableau, and the soul moves on into the next realm of the spiritual world, the soul realm.

Very young children, babies and toddlers, do not have this review. Their soul was still rooted in the spiritual world; they had not yet fully descended to earth. I often experience them as embedded, as 'links' between spiritual beings and human beings on earth. They do not leave their parents, one could say; they remain close to us.

Loving encounter

In the spiritual world we meet anew those with whom we were intimately connected on earth, in order that we may continue our life together, adapted to the circumstances there. Just as the soul lets go of everything it contained that was dependent on the physical body, in a similar way we are also freed of family connections that existed between people during earthly life. Thus we are no longer child, partner, parent, etc., we continue our life with the ones who were dear to us and with whom we had a spiritual bond, in a more profound connection than was possible on earth, in true, universal love. We understand each other better there than is possible on earth; we perceive the essential bond we have with each other.

We also meet those with whom we had conflicts. But in the spiritual world we can live with them in more profound connections than was possible on earth. We live through the things we did to each other and why we did them.

The more we have developed for ourselves during life on earth, the more insight we have gained there, the more we can perceive and understand in the spiritual world. We are our own lantern; we determine and order the light we ourselves radiate out.

Kamaloka

In the soul realm we process what was shown to us in the life tableau, beginning with the moment of death back to our birth. This realm is called kamaloka.* The journey of the soul through kamaloka is a path of detaching and processing. We take responsibility for our deeds on earth. We are not judged, we are not punished, but we reap what we have sown. Did we feel like part of creation, and did we live accordingly? How did we treat plants, animals and humans? Were we thankful for all that surrounded us? Did we always act with love and respect?

In the nights of our earthly life we always reflected on our past, present and future together with our guardian angel, whose task is to accompany the destiny of the individual human being, both before and after death. In the great review of our earthly life we look into our memories of these nights out of our higher consciousness – our I with whom we are now united again – and again our guardian angel helps us. In this review we experience the other as ourselves. This means that

---

* The word comes from Sanskrit. *Kama* means desire, longing; *loka* means place, only in reality it is not a place but a condition. In Catholicism the term *purgatory* is used.

we feel the joy we gave the other as our own joy, and the suffering we inflicted on the other as our own suffering.

Three thousand years before Christ, Krishna spoke: 'Thou art that. Thou art this other human being. How could you injure this other human being, for you injure yourself.'

Everything we did not want to accept or acknowledge during our life, we now perceive its justification, and we are able to view all events in their correct karmic relationships. We understand what we had to work out with others and why. And then the following arises in us, 'I want to set this right. Now only do I realise it; I am seeing it in a different light, shorn of sympathy and antipathy, retribution, injury, selfishness.'

What is also important and intriguing is that we can already do a great deal on earth in this regard. For instance, we can try to obtain insight in our own biography by writing the story of our life. Possibly we can then begin to see connections, and can have an inkling of why we experience one thing and another. This 'homework' helps us not only on earth, but also later in our kamaloka period.

Another important exercise is to try to discover the divine spark in our fellow humans and in ourselves, stripped of all outer qualities and aspects. It might lead us to try and straighten out our life and our relations with others; we can forgive and settle differences.

However, we might well take more good with us across the threshold than we thought. Nothing is lost of what we accomplished and created out of our will. Everything we brought about with love, great sacrifice and persistence, everything with which we were connected with heart and soul, has eternal value. And these are not always events for which we were praised on earth.

The connection of the dead with the earth

It often happens that people who had to say goodbye to a loved one are afraid that at a certain moment he or she will be 'completely gone.' This is a misunderstanding.

As long as the dead are dwelling in the soul realm they are very closely connected with the intimate family and friends of their completed life on earth. All they can remember, all that they are working through in kamaloka, is related to their fellow human beings. You can witness it in the mourning of those who were left behind; they too have many memories, and there is a reciprocal contact with the dead person. I often see this in my practice with mourning people; people become stuck in their mourning process, they are wrestling with something and then suddenly realise, as we are talking about it, that the bond is still there from both sides.

> The mutual understanding and love which unfolds here
> continues on into the regions of the spiritual world, even
> although, as the result of the one dying earlier, the other seems
> for a time to be separated from the dead. After this period
> has passed, the link that existed on earth is equally vital and
> intimate. The two are together, only all the purely natural,
> animal instincts must have been outlived. The feelings and
> thoughts which weave between one soul and another on earth
> are not hindered in yonder world by the encasements that exist
> here.
> – *Steiner*, Theosophy of the Rosicrucians, *May 29, 1907, p. 50*

Guided by higher beings we participate actively in the development of the earth after we have died. We assist the people on earth, depending on the capacities we have developed spiritually on earth.

Our further journey through the spiritual world

After a long, long time we leave the soul realm, of which kamaloka is but part. We move into other spheres, the true spirit realm, and learn much about genuine love, by which an ever deeper longing grows in us to fulfill the image that God created of the human being. The journey culminates when we go through what is called world midnight hour, where our true I beholds itself as it has become through many incarnations. It is an overwhelmingly lofty image, side by side with the image of the human being as intended to be when created. Out of a deep inner longing to live up to that image the resolution arises in us to return to the earth.

> As the days went past, Jonathan found himself thinking time and again of the Earth from which he had come. If he had known there just a tenth, just a hundredth, of what he knew here, how much more life would have meant! ... And the more Jonathan practised his kindness lessons, and the more he worked to know the nature of love, the more he wanted to go back to Earth.
> – *Bach*, Jonathan Livingston Seagull, *p. 60*

What follows on our journey is preparation for our return. We choose out of our higher I what we want to contribute to humanity in a following life, we collect the faculties we need to fulfill our destiny on earth, and we have a preview of that destiny. What we have not transformed in our prior life is taken up again for our next life.

What is heaven?

Writing this chapter – making the proper choices, finding the right words – has been a great struggle for me. For the great mystery cannot really be rendered in human language. Perhaps we can catch a radiance in our mirror, a glimpse of what is so inexpressible and far away, but which we human beings can sometimes, surprisingly and unexpectedly, sense to be so inexpressibly near our true home, the spiritual world. Because human language falls short I want to end the chapter with a picture I found in Richard Bach's book quoted above, *Jonathan*

Livingston Seagull, a fable-novella from the 1970s. The quotation begins
when Jonathan has died.

So this is heaven, he thought, and he had to smile at himself.
It was hardly respectful to analyse heaven in the very moment
that one flies up to enter it.

As he came from Earth now, above the clouds and in close
formation with the two brilliant gulls, he saw that his own body
was growing as bright as theirs. True, the same young Jonathan
Seagull was there that had always lived behind his golden eyes,
but the outer form had changed.

It felt like a seagull body, but already it flew far better
than his old one had ever flown. Why, with half the effort, he
thought, I'll get twice the speed, twice the performance of my
best days on earth!

His feathers glowed brilliant white now, and his wings
were smooth and perfect as sheets of polished silver. He began,
delightedly, to learn about them, to press power into these new
wings...

The clouds broke apart, his escorts called: 'Happy landings,
Jonathan,' and vanished into thin air.

He was flying over a sea, toward a jagged shoreline. A very
few seagulls were working the updrafts on the cliffs. Away off
to the north, at the horizon itself, flew a few others. New sights,
new thoughts, new questions...

The dozen gulls by the shoreline came to meet him, none
saying a word. He felt only that he was welcome and that
this was his home. It had been a big day for him, a day whose
sunrise he no longer remembered.

He turned to land on the beach, beating his wings to stop
an inch in the air, then dropping lightly to the sand. The other
gulls landed too, but none of them so much as flapped a feather.
They swung into the wind, bright wings outstretched, then

somehow they changed the curve of their feathers, until they had stopped in the same instant their feet touched the ground. It was beautiful control, but now Jonathan was just too tired to try it. Standing there on the beach, still without a word spoken, he was asleep.

In the days that followed, Jonathan saw that there was as much to learn about flight in this place as there had been in the life behind him. But with a difference. Here were gulls who thought as he thought. For each of them, the most important thing in living was to reach out and touch perfection in that which they most loved to do, and that was to fly. They were magnificent birds, all of them, and they spent hour after hour every day practising flight, testing advanced aeronautics.

For a long time Jonathan forgot about the world that he had come from, that place where the Flock lived with its eyes tightly shut to the joy of flight, using its wings as means to the end of finding and fighting for food. But now and then just for a moment, he remembered.

He remembered it one morning when he was out with his instructor, while they rested on the beach after a session of folded-wing snap rolls.

'Where is everybody, Sullivan?' he asked silently, quite at home now with the easy telepathy that these gulls used instead of screes and gracks. 'Why aren't there more of us here? Why, where I came from there were…'

'…thousands and thousands of gulls. I know.' Sullivan shook his head. 'The only answer I can see, Jonathan, is that you are pretty well a one-in-a-million bird. Most of us came along ever so slowly. We went from one world into another that was almost exactly like it, forgetting right away where we had come from, not caring where we were headed, living for the moment. Do you have any idea how many lives we must have gone through before we even got the first idea that there is more to life than eating, or fighting, or power in the Flock? A thousand lives, Jon, ten thousand! And then another hundred lives until we began to learn that there is such a thing as perfection, and another hundred again to get the idea that the purpose for living is to find that perfection and show it forth. The same rule holds for us now, of course: we choose our next world through what we learn in this one. Learn nothing, and the next world is the same as this one, all the same limitations and lead weights to overcome.'

One evening the gulls that were not night-flying stood together on the sand, thinking. Jonathan took all his courage in hand and walked to the Elder Gull who, it was said, was soon to be moving beyond this world.

'Chiang…' he said, a little nervously.

The old seagull looked at him kindly. 'Yes, my son?' Instead of being enfeebled by age, the Elder had been empowered by it; he could outfly any gull in the Flock, and he had learned the skills that the others were only gradually coming to know.

'Chiang, this world isn't heaven at all, is it?'

The Elder smiled in the moonlight. 'You are learning again, Jonathan Seagull,' he said.

'Well, what happens from here? Where are we going? Is there no such place as heaven?'

'No, Jonathan, there is no such place. Heaven is not a place, and it is not a time. Heaven is being perfect.'

– *Bach*, Jonathan Livingston Seagull, *pp. 51–54*

24

STAYING CONNECTED
WITH THE DEAD

We are not separated from the dead
By reality,
But by the limitations
Of our perception.

His name was Hans. We played together as toddlers and were in the same kindergarten. In high school we were in the same class again and had a close friendship. We did everything together, fell in love with the same girl, made a school journal together and had no secrets from each other.

Then he had an acute liver disease, wasted away in a few weeks and died due to complications. He was only 15.

To be this close to death was something I had never yet experienced. I couldn't grasp it. Intellectually I knew of course that he was dead, but my feelings told me that he wasn't. My inner experience was therefore not in step with outer reality. That confused me, and I had to think about it every day.

In the time that followed I began to see the world around me with very different eyes. Looking back, I would say that I began to experience the world in a spiritual manner, but at the time I had no words for it. Although I had been brought up with religion, in my environment these were completely unknown things. Therefore, I didn't speak about it with anyone. My mother says that I was very quiet at that time, which she ascribed to the passing of my friend. She let me be, for which I am still thankful.

After some time I got my new way of seeing things somewhat under control, but of course I still had many questions. Fortunately it was in the late 1960s when everyone was trying to expand their consciousness. Thus I was searching, trying things out, discovering things. In the end I landed on anthroposophy where I found words with which to clothe my experiences. I delved deeply into Steiner's books and noticed quite soon that my nightly dreams were beginning to change. My dreams had more structure and became more lucid and logical.

One night I was taken along up into the starry world by an angel. That felt familiar, but this time he took me much farther than previously. We went between the stars deep into the universe. There we arrived at a bright star. When we came close I saw the house where my friend had lived. Just as always I went around to the back and saw him standing in the yard. I recognised him right away, even though he had no physical form. He was like a star, a point of light emitting pulsating rays of light. The pulsation was like speaking; I recognised his voice.

Our reunion moved me deeply. I remembered that throughout the past five years I had always lived with the question of *why* he had died. The question welled up in me. To my surprise I noticed that I spoke in the same way he did. When I looked down I saw that my heart was also such a star. It made us laugh.

That night he really gave me the answer to my question. I cannot put that answer into words, but in my heart I fully understand it. When I woke up in the morning I felt freed of a heavy burden.

Today it is all decades ago, but I still feel a bond with the friend of my youth. When I think of him, as while writing these lines, I hear the sound of his voice and see the sparkle in his eye. That makes me happy and strong.

– *A friend of Hans*

I am grateful to Hans's friend for his story. The death of a friend at a young age is a radical event that can be like a watershed in life. It often takes a longer period of time before you realise that it perhaps also gives you much; it can give direction in your life, although I do not want to ignore the profound pain and desperation. It is important how you are supported and you and your grief are acknowledged.

Living with a question, carrying it with you inwardly, eventually leads you to an answer. Not a question about material well-being, but one about the meaning of things. If the question is also connected with a person who has died, it lays a 'foundation' for mutual contact.

I have often had the privilege of experiencing that when you can put your questions aside or on a backburner, patiently and in complete trust, the answers will come when you are ripe for them. Often they will come quite unexpectedly, even to the point that at the time you do not yet encompass the full significance. It may also happen that the answer falls into place with a bang, or reveals itself in a dream, an encounter in the night which you may remember.

Can the dead still mean something to us?

Because of my own experiences, my practice of many years, and all the talks with those who were left behind, I can answer this question with a whole-hearted yes. It is my conviction that the dead can and will virtually always, unconditionally, help us. We owe the dead much more than we perhaps realise. Our inspiration, our intuition, our ideas – do they all come from ourselves? Perhaps we are in a different world at night and are in loving contact with people who have died. The more we develop a sensitivity for this, the more this realm will open itself to us.

About ten years after the passing of my husband I suddenly had a feeling of 'Where are you now?' I said it aloud, alone in the room, from the bottom of my heart. That night I dreamed one of those dreams that is no dream, but an encounter you never forget. He showed me pictures of situations of myself and the children in the past ten years. I asked him: 'But how do you know all of that?' He lovingly replied: 'Of course I do, for I was with you all the time.' The question we ask the spiritual world to help us in our distress is audible there, and an audible question receives an answer human beings can comprehend.

Laura's father died after having lain in a coma for a number of days. She was eleven years old. Fifteen days after his death she met him:

> On a Friday afternoon I lay down on my bed for a moment, and suddenly I saw daddy standing before me! He lay down beside me and smiled. He said he had come out of the dark room and had seen how his life would have been if he had lived. That was not nice, he said; it was therefore better this way, and that he would always be with me. He also asked me if I would like to feel something: that the earth is turning. Of course I liked that! I said yes, and I really felt for twenty seconds that the earth was turning, and that was a great feeling! I wanted to say thank you, but he was already gone. So now I really know that this was absolutely the best way.
>
> I did not see him clearly all the time, but he was also a little transparent and had very beautiful eyes. I only saw his head, but the rest didn't interest me so much.

We learn to ask questions in deep distress and loneliness. Bearing our pain we become conscious of our inner shortcomings, we become aware of the limitations of our humanness. But it is also a stimulus toward inspiration, for when we become conscious of our shortcomings, we learn to ask questions, and these are the first steps toward inspiration. When we learn to understand the language that is spoken to us, the signs, the imagery, the so-called coincidences, the invisible half of our existence opens up, and a reciprocal contact becomes possible.

> My son was doing badly. I felt very, very sad and miserable, and went to the cemetery, to the grave of my mother. I put flowers

into a vase that is standing there and that she had given me, and said: 'Mom, I have so much sorrow, please help me.'

That evening I wanted to read the Bible to find some comfort. On the spur of the moment I took the old Bible I had received from my parents off the shelf. I leafed through it and suddenly found in the back in my mother's handwriting a reference to Matthew 11:28. I had never seen before that she had written that. I found the text: 'Come to me, all you who are weary and burdened, and I will give you rest.' I felt that she was very close to me and wanted to help me in my sorrow.

– Wilhelmina

Can we still mean something to the dead?

But what is the other side of the coin? Do those who have died still need us too? Do the dead also want to have contact with us? If that is so, what may it mean for a dead soul who wants to make contact with us, if we don't pick up the spiritual telephone or do not hear it ring? Have we even tried to build a telephone line? How could they ever reach us if we do not have any religious feelings or spiritual thoughts in us, or if we live with the idea that after death everything is finished? And immoral behaviour also makes a person on earth unreachable.

But when we bring true love to the dead and our fellow human beings and all that belongs to the creation, then we activate the contact with the dead. Love is a spiritual quality that is not stopped by the threshold of death. Love is the strength that makes the contact between the living and the dead possible, as well as contact with other spiritual beings. Not only do we badly need the dead, they need us just as much.

Someone who was very dear to me recently died, while he was under general anesthesia.

One evening he suddenly had a bad stomach pain. 'Just go home,' he said. 'I am no fun tonight, I had better be alone.'

The next morning he asked me to come and stay, for the pain had become virtually unbearable. We went to hospital emergency, for it was Sunday. We thought of stomach colic; the doctor suspected a stomach perforation. X-rays didn't show anything. The surgeon recommended exploratory surgery. Totally unexpectedly he was lying on an operating table within a half hour. The surgeon found an infection of the pancreas – life-threatening. They kept him under anesthesia to save his life forces so that the chance of recovery would be greater. Otherwise the pain would have been unbearable. He was hooked up to all kinds of equipment, including artificial respiration. After two and a half weeks he died while still under anesthesia.

Two weeks later I woke up in the middle of the night. There were images and a special atmosphere; I had to pay attention and listen carefully. And I knew: I have to grasp the meaning of it right away because once I am fully awake I will lose it. It worked.

The last two weeks of my friend's life had been touch and go. 'Am I going to make it or not? Will I survive or die? If I survive, how will I be, what will happen?' None of this – and it was a lot – could be shared with anyone. He said, 'I needed a body to tell it to others.' It was an enormous struggle, of rage and loneliness. He said: 'Those two and a half weeks were an eternity.'

He had wanted to share this with others, and this way it was perhaps still possible.

– *Christine*

We tend to think that the dead can 'see' everything, but perhaps things have to made visible for them too. It may happen that a dying person seeks contact with you at or around the moment of dying. When someone suddenly dies, for example due to an accident, it is possible that he or she is disoriented and looks for help.

My sister died suddenly in a traffic accident; it happened around midnight. I had just fallen asleep when with a start, between sleeping and waking, I sensed her presence. She was in a panic and asked for help.

'I don't know where I am, it is dark here!'

I asked: 'Can you see any light?'

'Yes, very far away.'

'Then go there, have confidence. You are not alone, stretch out your hands to the light, you can fly.'

I woke up, shaken, confused, but I had also seen a glimpse of light in the darkness. It had an attraction, but my sister needed a little push.

What on earth had happened? Why this fearful dream? It did not feel like a dream, but rather like reality. I got out of bed and couldn't sleep anymore. Unrest and fear oppressed me. Then the telephone rang. It was now two o'clock in the morning. Oh my God, I thought. It was my mother: 'Stephanie died in an accident.'

– *Elsa*

Sense of community

If we want to reach someone on earth we can call them on the phone, write a letter or email. But how do we seek contact with someone who has died?

When you enjoy something together with someone else in our world a sense of community arises. For instance, you watch a wonderful display of clouds, the white foam on the waves of a turbulent sea, a sunset or sunrise. You listen together to music or watch a sleeping child. These are moments of harmonious union between two human beings.

In the spiritual world we no longer have the senses we need for such experiences. But if on earth you intensely feel such moments again, the dead can participate in such feelings through soul contact.

No barrier can separate
What united in spirit preserves
The light-sparkling
And love-raying
Eternal soul bond.
As I am in your thoughts,
So may you be in mine.
– *Steiner,* 'For Georga Wiese' Our Dead, *p. 344*

We can also pray for the dead, speak a verse or read to them. Find a content with spiritual truth for this, such as the Bible, the Talmud, the Bhagavad Gita, anthroposophy, etc. The dead may not be able to literally hear the words and sounds we read to them, but they perceive where the text touches our heart, what lives in our thoughts. Our wonder and thankfulness for what is revealed to us from the spiritual realm is the bridge to the dead.

When we seek contact with a dead soul to whom we want to tell or read something, it helps to remember a moment that we intensely experienced together. We try to imagine it as exactly as we can, particularly what we felt then, what was happening, what the atmosphere was like. In other words, we experience it anew.

You don't so easily think of a quarrel. And yet, someone told me that he had had a vehement conflict with a colleague. He wanted to set that right after the person's death. He imagined the moment when the person hit the table with a thundering bang, and sensed that his colleague was immediately present.

You can also form a picture of someone's bearing, their gestures. How did they walk, what was the sound of their voice like? I can still hear how my daughter-in-law, who died aged 27, picked up the phone: 'Marina here!' Her young voice sparkled like little bells. Immediately she comes to life again for me.

I have often been told how people after a loved one had died had, to their own surprise, a certain idea or performed certain actions that had lived more in the consciousness of the person who had died than in their own, but which they had not been able to accomplish on earth. Because of these experiences a conviction has grown in me that it is possible for us to do all kinds of things on earth in place of people who have died.

Frequency

I am frequently asked by people how often they should read or say a verse. But in the spiritual world we do not live in time. In that world there is no time, only eternity. The concept of time only applies to the earth.

When in Wagner's opera, Parsifal enters the Grail Castle for the first time, he steps into a spiritual reality. Everything around him changes. He asks: 'Where am I?' The knight Gurnemanz replies: 'You see, my son, here time becomes space.' When we enter into the spiritual world time ceases to exist; it becomes space around you.

Rhythm, however, does seem to me to be important, both for here and for the other side. Rhythm brings health.

An elderly lady told me once that for years she had kept a 'death calendar' in which she noted the death days of family and friends. She would focus her attention on a person on the relative day and the night before. It had become a life task for her. In the course of time many of those living in the spiritual world would announce themselves already on the relative day which, for them, was their 'birthday.' Thus rhythm works as a cosmic experience of time.

But of course, a prayer or verse may also spontaneously well up from your heart at any time of day or night. Follow your intuition to sense what is genuine for your particular loved one. Don't let it become a duty. Find what is doable so you can stay within your own capacities; that gives you the strength to continue. Don't let yourself get fenced in by outer rules; don't imprison yourself.

Because at night we enter into dream consciousness, maybe the night could be a favourable time to ask a question of a loved one who has died.

A good time to prepare for this is when we are ready to fall asleep. Maybe we will receive an answer when we wake up, even though it will seem as if the answer came out of ourselves. Actually, we always fall asleep with a lot of questions, even though we are not conscious of it; and we are usually equally unconscious of the answers we receive. As we wake up it is important not to get into sense observations right away, but to try and remain a few moments in the realm where we came from.

It is self-evident that the question we ask must not contain any abstract thoughts from our materialistic life. Such thoughts do not reach the spiritual world. It has to be about questions of destiny or meaning, but also about a love or a deep longing to experience the being of another person. We might ask how we can help the other, or how we should understand the question of the other. It will, of course, take some time before we reach the point that we can understand the language of the dead and become able to make the right connection.

Meditation before falling asleep

Let all I have done
This day
Stand in the light
Of this night
That I may hear
What you are asking me
To think, to speak, to do.
Give that tomorrow,
Fumbling for your question
In the darkness of the day,
I find the courage
To think the truth,
To speak what's right,
To do the good.
– *Bastiaan Baan*

Meditation upon awakening

Every day
Has a hidden path
To a precious gift
Awaiting me.
Cautiously seeking,
Wakefully walking,
I grope my way
To the gift
Of this day.
– *Bastiaan Baan*

When you mourn a loved one you are completely filled with them. You are still so connected! Often you don't need to call up a picture, you are all memory. You know each other. The mutual connection is still so strong, only no longer tangible; you may feel as if amputated. Don't force yourself; nothing is mandatory, everything is allowed. Let your sorrow take its course; that is the bond of the soul. Your sorrow and despair are the price of your love. You have actually died a little also, but slowly you come back to earth.

Particularly in the first year, the dead may feel very close. However, the salutary numbness wears off, and the reality of 'never again' slowly becomes conscious. You feel lonely and abandoned. Never again will there be physical touch, never again visible communication. Thus in the course of years this arduous, so profoundly underestimated process shows many aspects. It is more than just grief; it may grow into an identity crisis. Your sense of value has changed; you have looked over the shoulder of the dead person and now you have to go it alone on earth. You have changed, but the world around you has not. It is a lonely road.

But still, the person who has died remains with you. At first they were your companion on earth, now they are a spectator. But when you begin to sense the influence and the interplay with the dead person, and understand it better, you become each other's companion again, but now on a different level. If that happens, you have received a gift. You stand closer to your intuition; in a certain way you have become clairvoyant, clair-feeling, clair-hearing.

A few years ago I was driving my car. I had to turn left after a stop sign and suddenly my dead husband was sitting next to me. In reflex I looked in my rearview mirror to check whether he had saved me from something, but there was no other traffic. It was wonderful. I didn't need to look beside me, he was simply there. Then I made the mistake that I wanted it to last a long time and hold on to it – but he slowly disappeared. A good lesson in case it happens again.

About a year after my father's death we were clearing out his things. It was a day of mourning. That evening I started with the preparations for a celebration in church on the first anniversary of his death. My father liked Toon Hermans [a Dutch comedian and writer] a lot, and I took a little book with his verses. I opened it at a verse about balloons that was just right for my father. I thought, 'Too bad, Dad, that we can't use a bunch of balloons in the celebration.'

A little later my mother came in. She had gone out on some errands and found two balloons by the front door, a red one and a white one. They had been blown our way; there was a carnival in town. I laughed inwardly and chuckled: 'Okay, Dad, but they are not complete. The colours of our town are red, white and yellow. First bring me the yellow one, then you will get your bunch of balloons in the church.'

A few hours later my husband came home from his work – with a yellow balloon in his hand! 'It was stuck against the front door!' Naturally we celebrated my father with a big bunch of balloons, and after the celebration we let them fly into the heights.

Sometime later I was looking for books in the library. I saw shelves with books about life after death. I caressed the books and thought: 'What is it like, Dad, to be dead?' He was instantly there. I felt him like an immense flame of burning love behind me. Motionless, without turning, I basked in his presence for more than a minute. Love, nothing but love.

It was as if he said, 'I love you,' and I whispered back, 'I love you too, Dad.'

– *Monique*

When we become conscious of the dead, we can rise in our soul above the daily worries that often so completely absorb us. Our consciousness changes, and this gives our daily life a different feeling. We learn to better distinguish between what is essential and what is not. That is the gift the dead give us.

Going together

Could it be the destiny of humanity that one day there will be unity again between human beings living on earth and the dead who live in the spiritual world? That we will be conscious again of the dead in our daily life? Presently there seems to be such a thick wall between here and there; the separation of a loved one is so painful, even though we know that they are with us. All that separates us from them is a veil of consciousness. May they live in our memory, not only as they were with us in the past, but in the here and now, standing behind me as I am writing this.

My inner gaze is on you.
I ardently wish that my love may warm you,
That I may sense your presence and inspiration,
That these may be woven into my daily life
So that our inner bond
May be mutual support
That we may fulfill
What lies in our destiny.

– *Renée Zeylmans*

AFTERWORD

If a shocking event takes place in your life that turns everything upside down, your life splits in two, as it were, and you often speak of before and after. That is what happened to me on April 30, 1974. We were driving in our old car to our vacation caravan in the countryside. It was about eleven in the morning, our three children of two, three and seven were in the back, the sun was shining pleasantly. I remember well that I felt so happy that I said a prayer of thanks, not knowing that two hours later my husband would suddenly die in the caravan. As modestly and gently as he always was, he slipped away from us. The children were there and said: 'Shh, Daddy is sleeping.'

Where in God's name do you find the strength to stay collected and bring the children to the restaurant of the manager of the place? There was at that moment but one thought: the children must not be left with trauma from this moment. I would never ever have been able to act the way I did without the help of the spiritual world. The sense that there was an angel who accompanied me was already strong when I was still a child, but after this event it was a certainty for me.

The death of my husband has given direction to my life. A few weeks after the funeral there was an intense inner moment; a prayer welled up in me: 'O God, if I ever get through this horror, this sorrow, let it then be meaningful for others who also have to go through this.'

I chose first to devote myself to bringing up the children. Fourteen years later, and after an intensive inner schooling, I was able to begin with my current work. It was preceded by another profound experience. Interestingly enough, on All Souls Day I was phoned because of a sudden death and had a very long phone call to support the family. When I finally put the phone down, another prayer rose up in me: 'O God, I feel that I can do this work, but show me the way.' I could hardly put up a sign saying: 'Mourners, come to me!' Deep within me a voice spoke: 'The dead will lead their loved ones to you.'

That's how it has indeed gone. Every year I thought that fewer people would knock on my door, but that was not so, on the contrary. It still surprises me, and I continue to look with wonder and gratitude to what is happening in my work. In the course of years I have given many lectures and workshops, and have taught in a variety of training programs. And soon my work also expanded to the weeks and months before dying.

And now my book is lying before you. Writing is a struggle for me. It is like composing music; a composer hears in their soul the great, heavenly sounds they want to bring out, but they have to squeeze them into notes on paper in order to put the music into the world. Similarly, what I wanted to put into my words first had to be condensed, and the reader has to bring it to life again.

As I was writing this book, I was time and again shown the way when I got stuck. The right people always crossed my path who could make a contribution to the book. Thank you all!

> The Road goes ever on and on,
> Down from the door where it began.
> Now far ahead the Road has gone,
> And I must follow, if I can,
> Pursuing it with eager feet,
> Until it joins some larger way
> Where many paths and errands meet.
> And whither then? I cannot say.
> – *Tolkien,* The Fellowship of the Ring, *I.1*

FURTHER READING

Care for the dying

Bentheim, Tineke van, *Home Nursing for Carers,* Floris Books, UK 2006. A comprehensive guide to holistic home care for those nursing children and adults through an illness, including nursing the terminally ill.

Death and dying

Baum, John, *When Death Enters Life,* Floris Books, UK 2003. Experiences, observations and practical advice enabling those encountering death to meet it in an active manner, both mentally and physically.

Bockemühl, Almut, *The Twilight Years: Thoughts on Old Age, Death and Dying,* Temple Lodge, UK 2016.

Drake, Stanley, *Though you Die: Death and Life Beyond Death,* free PDF from www.florisbooks.co.uk

Kübler-Ross, Elisabeth, *On Death and Dying: What the Dying have to teach Doctors, Nurses, Clergy and their own Families,* Scribner, USA 1969.

Wijnberg, Nicholas and Philip Martyn, *Crossing the Threshold,* Temple Lodge, UK 2003. Practical and spiritual guidance on death and dying.

Near-death experiences

Moody, Raymond, *Life after Life,* Mockingbird, USA 1975. One of the first books on near-death experiences.

Platt, Adam, *A Rainbow over the River: Experiences of Life, Death and Other Worlds,* Clairview, UK.

Roszell, Calvert, *The Near-Death Experience,* Lindisfarne Books, USA 2019. An insightful study into near-death experience, drawing on the work of Michael Sabom and Rudolf Steiner.

Funerals

Baum, John, *Rituals around Death,* free PDF from www.florisbooks.co.uk

The afterlife

Brink, Margarete van den, and Hans Stolp, *What Happens When we Die? Our Journey in the Afterlife,* Temple Lodge, UK 2017.

Childs, Gilbert, *The Journey Continues: Finding a New Relationship to Death,* Rudolf Steiner Press, UK 1999. Finding a new relationship to death by considering the journey beyond.

Kübler-Ross, Elisabeth, *On Life after Death,* Celestial Arts, USA 1984.

Steiner, Rudolf, *Death as Metamorphosis of Life* (CW 182) SteinerBooks, USA 2008.

—, *Life Beyond Death,* Rudolf Steiner Press, UK 1995.

Grieving, mourning

Kübler-Ross, Elisabeth, and David Kessler, *On Grief and Grieving,* Simon & Schuster, USA 2005.

Ploeger, Maarten, *Honeymoon of Mourning,* Adonis Press, USA 2016. A beautiful and moving collection of ninety poems around the themes of death, separation and bereavement.

Meditations and connection to the dead

Blatchford, Claire, *Experiences with the Dying and the Dead: Waking to Our Connections with Those Who Have Died,* Lindisfarne Books, USA 2007. Explores the threshold between life and death through a series of personal stories.

Heisler, Hermann, *Our Relationship to Those Who Have Died,* Steiner College Press, USA.

Stedall, Jonathan, *No Shore Too Far: Meditations on Death, Bereavement and Hope,* Hawthorn Press, UK 2017.

Steiner, Rudolf, *The Connection between the Living and the Dead* (CW 168), SteinerBooks, USA 2017.

—, *Life Between Death and Rebirth: The Active Connection Between the Living and the Dead* (CW140) Anthroposophic Press, USA 1975.

—, *Meditations for the Dead,* Rudolf Steiner Press, UK 2018.

—, *The Presence of the Dead on the Spiritual Path,* Anthroposophic Press, USA 1990.

—, *Staying Connected: How to Continue your Relationship with Those Who Have Died,* Anthroposophic Press, USA 1999.

Death of children

Mathes, Charlotte, *And a Sword Shall Pierce Your Hearth: Moving from Despair to Meaning after the Death of a Child,* Chiron, USA.

Schilling, Karin, *Where Are You? Coming to Terms with the Death of My Child,* Anthroposophic Press, USA 1988.

Suicide, euthanasia

Hamdi, Nabeel, *Life Beyond the Darkness: The Healing of a Suicide Across the Threshold of Death,* Clairview, UK 2000.

Prokofieff, Sergei and Peter Selg, *Honoring Life: Medical Ethics and Physician-Assisted Suicide,* SteinerBooks, USA 2015. A consideration from an anthroposophical point of view.

Stajano, Attilio, *Only Love Remains: Lessons from the Dying on the Meaning of Life – Euthanasia or Palliative Care?* Clairview, UK 2015.

Books quoted in the text

Bach, Richard, *Jonathan Livingston Seagull,* Macmillan, USA 1970.

Bhagavad Gita, The, tr. Laurie L. Patton, Penguin Classics 2008.

Beckh, Hermann, *Alchymie: Vom Geheimnis der Stoffeswelt,* Dornach 1987.

Bittleston, Adam, *Prayers and Meditative Verses.*

Bomans, Godfried, *Sprookjes van Godfried Bomans* [Fairytales] Amsterdam 1990.

Dalai Lama, *Open Heart, Clear Mind,* Snow Lion 1990.

Debus, Michael, *Begleitung über den Tod hinaus,* Gesundheit Aktiv 2000.

Douglas-Klotz, Neil, *Prayers of the Cosmos: Meditations on the Aramaic Words of Jesus,* HarperCollins 1994.

Du hast mich heimgesucht bei Nacht. Abschiedsbriefe und Aufzeichnungen des Widerstandes 1933–1945, [You plagued me by night. Farewell letters and writings of the resistance] published by Helmut Gollwitzer, Käthe Kuhn and Reinhold Schneider, Munich.

Dyke, Henry van, *The Story of the Other Wise Man,* Harper & Row.

Eeden, Frederik van, *Pauls ontwaken* [Paul's awakening] Katwijk 1983.

Eichendorff, Joseph von, (1788-1857), *Moon Night.*

Eijck, P.N. van, *Herwaarts,* Haarlem 1939.

Emmichoven, J. E. Zeylmans van, *Who was Ita Wegman, A Documentation,* Vol. I, Mercury Press 1995.

Frieling, Rudolf, *Im Zeichen der Hoffnung,* Stuttgart 1986.

Gibran, Kahlil, *The Prophet,* Alfred A. Knopf, 2002.

Hahn, Herbert, et al., *Wir erlebten Rudolf Steiner.*

Hammarskjöld, Dag, *Markings,* Alfred A. Knopf 1973.

Hofacker, Erich P. *Christian Morgenstern,* Twayne Publishers 1978.

Jonas, Hans, *The Concept of God after Auschwitz,* Journal of Religion (67:1) 1987.

Lindholm, Dan, *Encounters with Angels,* Floris Books 1993.

Morse, Melvin, *Closer to the Light,* Random House 1990.

Osis, Karlis, and Erlendur Haraldsson, *At the Hour of Death,* Time Life 1993.

Rinpoche, Sogyal, *Glimpse after Glimpse, Daily Reflections on Living and Dying.* Rider.

—, *The Tibetan Book of Living and Dying,* HarperCollins e-book.

Saint-Exupéry, Antoine de, *The Little Prince,* Harcourt, Brace & World 1943.

Sheldrake, Rupert, *The Sense of Being Stared At,* Hutchinson 2003.

Solomon, Lewis D. *The Jewish Book of Living and Dying,* Jason Aronson, 1999.

Steiner, Rudolf. Volume Nos refer to the Collected Works (CW), or to the German Gesamtausgabe (GA).

—, *Karmic Relationships,* Vol. II (CW 236) Rudolf Steiner Press, UK 1974.

—, *Initiation Science and the Development of the Human Mind* (CW 228) Rudolf Steiner Press, UK 2016.

—, *Spiritual Life Now and after Death* (CW 157a) SteinerBooks, USA 2013.

—, *Theosophy* (CW 9) Anthroposophic Press, USA 1994.

—, *Theosophy of the Rosicrucian* (CW 99) Rudolf Steiner Press, UK 1981.

—, *Verses and Meditations* (part of GA 40) Rudolf Steiner Press, UK 2004.

Stolp, Hans, *Als dood te vroeg komt* [When death comes too early], Kampen 1987.

Tagore, Rabindranath, *Gitanjali: Songs of Offering,* 1910.

—, *The Heart of God,* Tuttle, USA 1997.

Tolkien, J.R.R. *The Fellowship of the Ring,* Houghton Mifflin 1965.

Wegener, Dagny, *Blick in eine andere Welt. Begegnungen mit Verstorbenen und geistigen Wesen,* Stuttgart 1997.

Zajonc, Arthur, *Catching the Light,* Bantam Books 1993.

Zeylmans van Emmichoven, *see* Emmichoven, J. E. Zeylmans van

CONTRIBUTORS

Bastiaan Baan is a priest of the Christian Community working in the Netherlands and recently as seminary director in USA. He is author of a number of books on Christian spirituality.

Toke Bezuijen is a carer and specialist in external therapies like compresses, baths and rhythmic massage.

Hilly Bol studied music therapy in Montana, USA, and works at a hospice in Rotterdam.

Pauli van Engelen is a carer and specialist in external therapies like compresses, baths and rhythmic massage.

Marieke Udo de Haes-Mulder is an art therapist who lectured at Leiden.

Paul Schmitz is a physician in a care home on Bilthoven, Netherlands.

Bert Voorhoeve gives courses and workshops on the imagery of fairytales through retelling, painting and acting.

Patricia de Vos is a psychologist at the University Children's Hospital in Ghent, Belgium.

Monique van der Zanden is an author of children's books.